This book is intended as a reference volume only, not as a medical manual.
The information given here is designed to help you make informed decisions about your health.
It is not intended as a substitute for any treatment that may have been prescribed by your doctor.
If you suspect that you have a medical problem, we urge you to seek competent medical help.

The information in this book is meant to supplement, not replace, proper exercise training.
All forms of exercise pose some inherent risks. The editors and publisher advise readers to take full
responsibility for their safety and know their limits. Before practicing the exercises in this book,
be sure that your equipment is well-maintained, and do not take risks beyond your level of experience,
aptitude, training, and fitness. The exercise and dietary programs in this book are not intended as
a substitute for any exercise routine or dietary regimen that may have been prescribed by your doctor.
As with all exercise and dietary programs, you should get your doctor's approval before beginning.

Mention of specific companies, organizations, or authorities in this book
does not imply endorsement by the author or publisher, nor does mention of specific companies,
organizations, or authorities imply that they endorse this book, its author, or the publisher.

Internet addresses and telephone numbers given in this book were accurate at the time it went to press.

© 2017 by Hearst Magazines, Inc.

Women's Health® is a registered trademark of Hearst Magazines, Inc.

Printed in China

Photographs by Ryan Orlowski

Book design by Laura White

ISBN: 978-1-95009-909-2

10 paperback

HEARST

CONTENTS

LET'S GET STRONG!

Women are made to be strong. Energetic. Capable. Our bodies are intended to take us wherever we want to go in life—whether that's up Mt. Kilimanjaro, through the Boston Marathon finish line, or onto an airplane without needing help with our overhead bags. None of that happens without strength. It's what allows us to live at our full potential.

As a certified personal trainer, Nike Master Trainer, and, now, the 2017 *Women's Health* Next Fitness Star, I've felt the freedoms that strength affords—as well as the limitations that come with being, well, not so physically strong.

Growing up as a dancer, and playing professionally in a cover band in my twenties, I was always aerobically fit, and assumed that meant I was "in good shape." But dancing on stage with a bass slung over my shoulder each night took a toll on my body. I felt constantly run-down, sore, and sapped for energy. I thought that was natural—until I took my first one-on-one strength training class with a personal trainer. I was shocked to realize how little muscular strength I actually had!

I immediately set my sights on getting strong, and as I trained, I realized how much better it made me feel—in body and mind. I had more energy. I didn't ache like I used to. As I became more confident in the gym and in my body, that attitude permeated every area of my life. I felt invincible. If I could pull my body over a pullup bar, squat my bodyweight, and rock a one-handed pushup, what couldn't I do? I wanted other people to feel that way, too. I became a certified personal trainer and, for six years, my mission has been to help other women live fully by developing their own strength.

HOW THIS PROGRAM WORKS

Strength doesn't come from doing things that are easy. By taking on incrementally greater challenges in the gym—a process referred to as progressive overload—your body gets stronger and better equipped to perform those challenges. Then you take on new challenges—ones that are just tough enough to keep your body progressing and growing.

That's why following an exercise plan like this one is so important. By taking you through 12 weeks of consistent and progressive resistance workouts, this program will help you build a base of strength and get started on your own lifelong fitness journey. The possibilities of where it will take you are endless.

Want to look lean and toned? Strength training helps you burn fat while maintaining your muscles, giving you a badass, fit-looking body. (Check out page 12 to learn more about lifting for fat loss and why you shouldn't worry about getting "bulky"!) More importantly, studies show that lifting helps women develop healthy body images. You'll start to appreciate what your body can do—not just how it looks.

If you want to perform 10 pushups in a row, squat a barbell loaded with your full bodyweight, or rock your first chinup, get excited! This program will help get you there. You'll notice a difference outside the gym, too. Carrying groceries and climbing stairs gets easier. You'll walk with more confidence. These results don't happen overnight, but after 12 weeks of work, you can expect to be stronger, fitter, and well on your way to crushing your goals. Stick with it for a lifetime, and you'll lead a longer, healthier life.

This 12-week program is divvied up into three four-week stages, with each stage building on the last one to continually challenge your body, prevent plateaus, and keep things fun! You can find more details in the pages to come, but here's the gist:

STAGE 1

Build a foundation, learn proper form, and strengthen your body in the seven basic movement patterns.

STAGE 2

Integrate bigger compound lifts, increase weights, and decrease reps to improve total-body strength and stability.

STAGE 3

Focus on heavy barbell lifts to build serious strength.

Within each stage, you'll rotate through four weekly workouts: Workout 1, Workout 2, Workout 3, and Workout 4. Schedule your workouts on the days that are most convenient for you, but try not to take more than two days off in a row. You can perform the workouts on back-to-back days, but make sure to give yourself at least one day of recovery after two or three workouts in a row.

Recovery days give your muscles the time they need to repair and grow stronger from your workouts. A light recovery workout—like yoga, moderate cardio, foam rolling, or Pilates—can actually aid this process by getting your blood flowing to your muscles, promoting repair. But that's optional—you can simply rest on your recovery days, too.

Workout Structure

WARMUP

Each workout begins with a very brief warmup. This is just as important as any other part of your workout. You'll do one mobility exercise, which increases your range of motion in key joints that you'll use in that workout. And you'll do one activation exercise, which "wakes up" and primes the muscles that you're about to work.

Perform both exercises for the prescribed number of reps, then repeat for a total of two sets of each exercise. If you feel like you need to complete three or more sets to really wake up your muscles, go for it!

CIRCUIT

These are your four main strength-building exercises. Perform them as a circuit: Complete the prescribed number of reps of the first exercise (labeled 2A on the workout page), then move on to the other three exercises in the circuit (labeled 2B, 2C, and 2D) with little to no rest between moves. Once you've completed one set of all four exercises, rest for 1 to 2 minutes. That's one round. Repeat until you have completed the prescribed number of sets of each exercise.

SUPERSET

You'll finish your workout with a superset of two exercises designed to supplement your main strength circuit, combining total-body, core, stability, and isolation moves. Perform each exercise for the amount of reps suggested, with little to no rest between the movements. After completing both exercises, rest for 1 to 2 minutes. That's one round. Repeat one time for a total of two sets of each exercise.

What You'll Need

The workouts utilize basic equipment you can find in most gyms.

☐ FULL RANGE OF DUMBBELLS

☐ CABLE MACHINES WITH HIGH, LOW, AND IN-BETWEEN SETTINGS, ALONG WITH STIRRUP, ROPE, AND LAT BAR ATTACHMENTS (if you don't know what those are, you'll see them in the photos that correspond with each exercise)

☐ FLAT AND ADJUSTABLE BENCHES

☐ MINIBAND AND RESISTANCE BAND

☐ SQUAT RACK OR POWER RACK WITH BARBELL, FULL RANGE OF WEIGHT PLATES, AND WEIGHT CLIPS (to keep your weight plates secure on the barbell)

☐ YOGA MAT

☐ TOWEL

☐ STOPWATCH OR TIMER

If you're working out at home, on the road, or in a crowded gym, some of the equipment above may not be available. No worries—the workouts in this program can be tailored to fit the equipment on hand, as long as you have dumbbells. Look up the problem move in the exercise guide and find a similar exercise from the same movement pattern (more on that on page 10) that you can substitute in. For example, if your workout includes a barbell front squat but you don't have a barbell, do a goblet squat instead. Another idea that works well for crowded gyms is to skip the problem move in your circuit and do it later as a straight set. That is, do all sets of the same move in a row—resting 1 to 2 minutes between sets—once the equipment becomes available.

TRACK YOUR PROGRESS

The following challenges will test your strength in key muscle groups that are about to get *a lot* stronger. Perform each of the challenges before beginning the program and jot down your results. (Each of the moves are fully described in the exercise guide starting on page 44.)

Then repeat the test at the end of each workout stage.

Even if you're not proud of your Week 1 results, trust me: By Week 12, you'll be very glad to have a record of where you started and how far you've come. One of the best feelings in the world is making real, concrete progress in what your body can do. And when you're banging out 10 full pushups with ease, it can be hard to remember a time when you could barely do one! This chart is proof of your hard work.

How many reps of these exercises can you complete in 1 minute?

EXERCISE	WEEK 1	WEEK 4	WEEK 8	WEEK 12
Hand-Release Pushup PAGE 92				
Prisoner Squat PAGE 70				
Inverted Row PAGE 102				

How long can you perform these exercises?
(If you hit 1 minute, you've maxed out!)

EXERCISE	WEEK 1	WEEK 4	WEEK 8	WEEK 12
Farmer's Carry (30-lb Dumbbells) PAGE 108				
Hollow-Body Hold PAGE 57				
Side Plank (Right) PAGE 59				
Side Plank (Left) PAGE 59				

STRENGTH TRAINING 101

How To Choose The Right Weight

Finding the right weights involves some trial and error, even for experienced lifters. So don't worry! Always guess light. If you end the set feeling like you have more than one or two good reps left in you, that's your cue to increase your weight on the next set. Make a note of your weights as you go, which will help you home in on your ideal number. (This workout plan includes space to track your weights—use it!)

The Right Way To Breathe

Deep, diaphragmatic breathing, also called belly breathing, helps you move better and efficiently get oxygen to your muscles. Focus on slowly inhaling so that your belly expands as you move through the eccentric, or easy, part of an exercise. Then, forcefully exhale through your mouth to tighten your core as you move into the concentric, or difficult, part of an exercise. (Put another way, the concentric part is where you're pushing or pulling. For example, when you're pulling the bar to your chest in a lat pulldown or pushing your body up in a pushup.)

An Important Note On Tempo

Unless otherwise instructed, do all exercises with a 2-1-1 count. That means you'll perform the eccentric part of the exercise over the course of two seconds, hold for one second, and perform the concentric part over the course of one second. For example, in a lunge, lower toward the floor for two seconds, hold for one, and then rise back up in one.

Some exercises are marked as "tempo," like the Tempo Incline Pushup. For those moves, use a 4-1-1 count. Perform the eccentric part slowly over the course of four seconds, hold for one, then perform the concentric part over the course of one second.

The 7 Movement Patterns

All movements—not just in the gym, but in everyday life—can be broken down into seven fundamental patterns. Simply put, they are the seven ways in which our bodies are designed to move. Any strength program should (and this one will!) improve your body's ability to move through these patterns, both in and out of the weight room.

SQUAT

Most women think squats mean booty, booty, booty. While squats *are* great for strengthening your glutes—your body's largest muscle group—they also train your quadriceps, hamstrings, and important stabilizer muscles throughout your core. This movement pattern, which involves moving through both the knee and hip joints, is to thank every time you get up out of a chair or bend down to pick something up off the floor.

HIP HINGE

The hip hinge is all about moving your hips through their full range of motion. By doing so, exercises such as glute bridges, hip thrusts, and deadlifts train the muscles that make up your posterior chain (your body's backside) in a big way. They focus in on your hamstrings and all-important glutes.

PUSH

Pushups, chest presses, and overhead shoulder presses are the most common ways we perform pushing movements in the gym. Prepare to strengthen your chest, shoulders, and triceps and become better at throwing and punching. Hey, every woman should know self-defense!

PULL

Pulling exercises—including rows and pullups—are incredibly important for everyday function. Performing them strengthens your back to combat the aches, pains, and postural problems associated with working on computers, tablets, and phones all day. Sculpted biceps are another bonus.

LUNGE

Every time you walk, jog, or run, you are performing a variation of a lunge—moving your body's weight from one foot to another. Strengthening each leg's glutes, quads, and hamstrings separately, lunges also improve total-body balance and core stability.

CARRY

Pick up something heavy and walk. This simple movement pattern is fundamental to our daily lives—from lugging huge purses to moving furniture. Performing carry variations in the weight room makes you significantly stronger all over, but especially improves your core and grip strength. Both become increasingly important as you lift heavier.

ROTATION

Rotation is one of the most underrated, yet necessary movement patterns your body performs on a daily basis. Every day, whether you're swinging a bat or reaching behind you into the back seat of your car, you're rotating in some way. This program trains you to become stronger when you move rotationally—not just up and down and forward and backward.

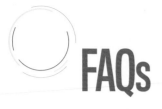

FAQs

I feel self-conscious at the gym. How do I get more comfortable?

Everyone feels that way when starting out! But it doesn't last long. If you feel awkward the first time you use a new piece of equipment or try out a new exercise, remind yourself that simply learning this stuff is progress. You just have to get through a few uncomfortable workouts, and then you'll be banging out reps like a boss. Promise.

In the meantime, ask a friend with similar exercise goals to go to the gym with you. A workout partner can help you feel more confident—even if you're both beginners. You can also try carving out a less-public corner of your gym to lift in, like an empty group fitness room, so you don't feel like you're on display. Or try visiting the gym at non-peak hours when it's not so crowded.

Will lifting heavy weights make me bulky?

Building big muscles is a lot harder than most people assume. Adding size requires targeted training and nutrition. For women, that's especially true. We simply don't have the testosterone levels needed to pack on muscle to the same degree that men do. Yes, I've designed this program to help you build *some* muscle. But if you're concerned about getting "bulky," rest assured that a pound of muscle takes up less space than a pound of fat. As you build muscle and burn fat, your body measurements will actually decrease. And since building muscle doesn't happen overnight, you'll have plenty of time to adjust your training if you think you've put on enough muscle. Meanwhile, if you are interested in significantly increasing muscle size, this plan will help you build the strength basis needed to reach your goals in the future.

Is strength training going to help me lose weight?

It's time to dispel the myth that, if you want to lose fat, you should spend all (or even most!) of your time on cardio machines. Harvard research even shows that, minute per minute, strength training is better at warding off abdominal fat—which is largely to blame for chronic obesity-related conditions such as heart disease and insulin resistance—compared to cardio. That's because, unlike cardio, which leads to weight loss from both fat and muscle, strength training zeroes in on fat. It maintains and builds your muscle, which is your metabolism's driving force, helping you burn more calories both in and out of the gym.

A note about your weight: It's easy to get caught up in the scale, but it's not the best marker of progress, especially when it comes to strength training. Remember that this program is designed to help you build muscle while you lose fat. So it's possible that even if you're losing fat, your weight won't change significantly. You may even see yourself gaining some weight from added muscle, and that's OK!

Instead of worrying about your weight, track your progress with the strength test on page 8. Also consider keeping tabs on other measurements like body composition (many electronic scales now measure body fat percentage) or waist circumference, instead of fixating on the one number on the scale.

What should I do if an exercise is too difficult?

It's important to always perform exercises with proper form. So, if you cannot use proper form, do an easier variation of the move. Don't feel discouraged—as long as you're challenging yourself, you're making progress. The simplest way to make an exercise easier is to decrease the resistance used, whether that means using a lighter dumbbell or doing a modified pushup with your hands elevated instead of a traditional one. Refer to the exercise guide (page 44) for ideas on how to modify, or just continue doing an easier variation from earlier in the program.

What should I do if something hurts?

If you feel pain in a joint or a sharp pain in a muscle, stop what you are doing immediately. Do not push through pain or something that "just doesn't feel right." Consider talking to a trainer, physical therapist, or sports medicine doctor about why a given movement hurts and what you can do about it. In the meantime, skip the problem move until you can do it without pain. The exercise variations included in the exercise guide (page 44) will also help you tailor the moves to work around cranky joints or prior injuries.

Should I train when I'm still store?

Delayed onset muscle soreness, that ache you get in your muscles 24 to 72 hours after a workout, is a natural part of performing a new exercise or going up in weight. These workouts are designed so that you can perform them on back-to-back days, so it's likely that, every now and then, you will work out while you're a little sore. That's perfectly fine. But if every single move hurts or the soreness is keeping you from moving like you usually would, it's best to call it a recovery day.

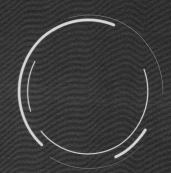

STAGE ONE

The first four weeks of this program are all about building a strong foundation for the weeks to come. You'll strengthen your body as it moves through the seven basic movement patterns and master proper form and technique. Many movements work each side of your body separately to help you learn proper form without the extra coordination required when performing bilateral (two-sided) movements. Also, many overhead movements occur from seated or kneeling positions to help you avoid using your lower body to generate momentum. All workouts take about 30 minutes.

STAGE 1 > WORKOUT 1

WARMUP > 2 SETS

1A Side-Lying Shoulder Sweep
15 REPS

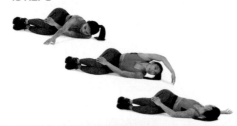

1B Plank
30 SECONDS

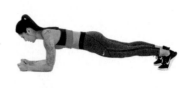

CIRCUIT > 3 SETS

2A Tempo Incline Pushup
10–12 REPS

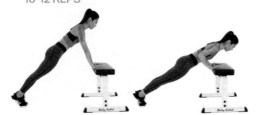

2B Single-Arm Row
10–12 REPS

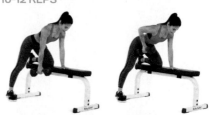

2C Seated Alternating Overhead Press
10–12 REPS

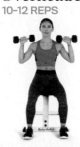

2D Single-Arm Half-Kneeling Lat Pulldown
10–12 REPS

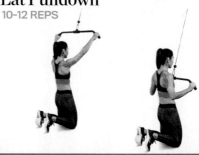

SUPERSET > 2 SETS

3A Farmer's Carry
30 REPS

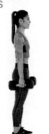
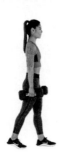

3B Plank with Alternating Hip Dip
10 REPS

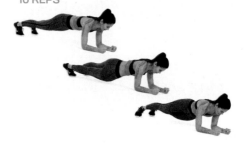

STAGE 1 > WORKOUT 1 > LOG

Use this space to record how much weight you use and how many reps you complete on each set. This will help you select the right weights and track your progress from week to week.

1A Side-Lying Shoulder Sweep

WEEK	REPS	SET 1	SET 2
1	15		
2	15		
3	15		
4	15		

1B Plank

WEEK	REPS	SET 1	SET 2
1	30 seconds		
2	30 seconds		
3	30 seconds		
4	30 seconds		

2A Tempo Incline Pushup

WEEK	REPS	SET 1	SET 2	SET 3
1	10-12			
2	10-12			
3	10-12			
4	10-12			

2B Single-Arm Row

WEEK	REPS	SET 1	SET 2	SET 3
1	10-12			
2	10-12			
3	10-12			
4	10-12			

2C Seated Alternating Overhead Press

WEEK	REPS	SET 1	SET 2	SET 3
1	10-12			
2	10-12			
3	10-12			
4	10-12			

2D Single-Arm Half-Kneeling Lat Pulldown

WEEK	REPS	SET 1	SET 2	SET 3
1	10-12			
2	10-12			
3	10-12			
4	10-12			

3A Farmer's Carry

WEEK	REPS	SET 1	SET 2
1	30		
2	30		
3	30		
4	30		

3B Plank with Alternating Hip Dip

WEEK	REPS	SET 1	SET 2
1	10		
2	10		
3	10		
4	10		

STAGE 1 > WORKOUT 2

WARMUP > 2 SETS

1A Alternating Lateral Squat
15 REPS

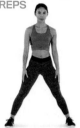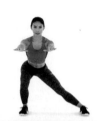

1B Miniband Squat
15 REPS

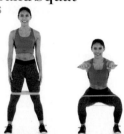

CIRCUIT > 3 SETS

2A Tempo Goblet Squat
10–12 REPS

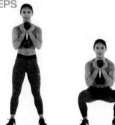

2B Dumbbell Glute Bridge
10–12 REPS

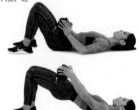

2C Alternating Dumbbell Reverse Lunge
10–12 REPS

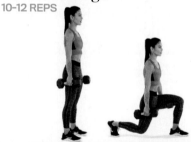

2D Dumbbell Sumo Deadlift
10–12 REPS

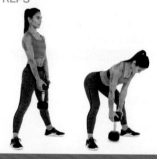

SUPERSET > 2 SETS

3A Alternating Lateral Bound
15 REPS

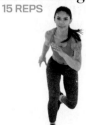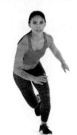

3B Bodyweight Hamstring Curl
15 REPS

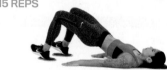
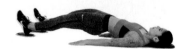

STAGE 1 > WORKOUT 2 > LOG

Use this space to record how much weight you use and how many reps you complete on each set. This will help you select the right weights and track your progress from week to week.

1A Alternating Lateral Squat

WEEK	REPS	SET 1	SET 2
1	15		
2	15		
3	15		
4	15		

1B Miniband Squat

WEEK	REPS	SET 1	SET 2
1	15		
2	15		
3	15		
4	15		

2A Tempo Goblet Squat

WEEK	REPS	SET 1	SET 2	SET 3
1	10-12			
2	10-12			
3	10-12			
4	10-12			

2B Dumbbell Glute Bridge

WEEK	REPS	SET 1	SET 2	SET 3
1	10-12			
2	10-12			
3	10-12			
4	10-12			

2C Alternating Dumbbell Reverse Lunge

WEEK	REPS	SET 1	SET 2	SET 3
1	10-12			
2	10-12			
3	10-12			
4	10-12			

2D Dumbbell Sumo Deadlift

WEEK	REPS	SET 1	SET 2	SET 3
1	10-12			
2	10-12			
3	10-12			
4	10-12			

3A Alternating Lateral Bound

WEEK	REPS	SET 1	SET 2
1	15		
2	15		
3	15		
4	15		

3B Bodyweight Hamstring Curl

WEEK	REPS	SET 1	SET 2
1	15		
2	15		
3	15		
4	15		

STAGE 1 > WORKOUT 3

WARMUP > 2 SETS

1A Bird Dog
10 REPS

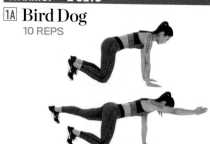

1B Prone Shoulder Squeeze
15 REPS

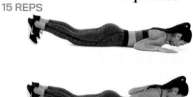

CIRCUIT > 3 SETS

2A Tempo Dumbbell Bent-Over Row
10–12 REPS

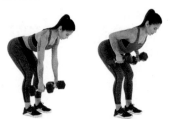

2B Bridge Hold with Dumbbell Chest Press
10–12 REPS

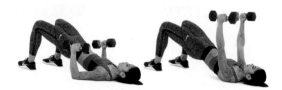

2C Inverted Row
10–12 REPS

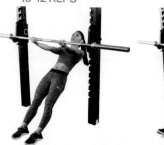
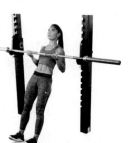

2D Half-Kneeling Low-to-High Dumbbell Chop
10–12 REPS

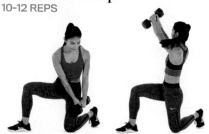

SUPERSET > 2 SETS

3A Plank with Alternating Leg Lift
10 REPS

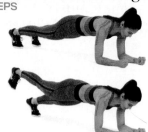

3B Hollow-Body Hold
20–60 SECONDS

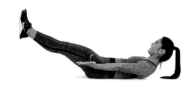

STAGE 1 > WORKOUT 3 > LOG

Use this space to record how much weight you use and how many reps you complete on each set. This will help you select the right weights and track your progress from week to week.

1A Bird Dog

WEEK	REPS	SET 1	SET 2
1	10		
2	10		
3	10		
4	10		

1B Prone Shoulder Squeeze

WEEK	REPS	SET 1	SET 2
1	15		
2	15		
3	15		
4	15		

2A Tempo Dumbbell Bent-Over Row

WEEK	REPS	SET 1	SET 2	SET 3
1	10-12			
2	10-12			
3	10-12			
4	10-12			

2B Bridge Hold with Dumbbell Chest Press

WEEK	REPS	SET 1	SET 2	SET 3
1	10-12			
2	10-12			
3	10-12			
4	10-12			

2C Inverted Row

WEEK	REPS	SET 1	SET 2	SET 3
1	10-12			
2	10-12			
3	10-12			
4	10-12			

2D Half-Kneeling Low-to-High Dumbbell Chop

WEEK	REPS	SET 1	SET 2	SET 3
1	10-12			
2	10-12			
3	10-12			
4	10-12			

3A Plank with Alternating Leg Lift

WEEK	REPS	SET 1	SET 2
1	10		
2	10		
3	10		
4	10		

3B Hollow-Body Hold

WEEK	REPS	SET 1	SET 2
1	20-60 seconds		
2	20-60 seconds		
3	20-60 seconds		
4	20-60 seconds		

STAGE 1 > WORKOUT 4

WARMUP > 2 SETS

1A Groin Rock
10 REPS

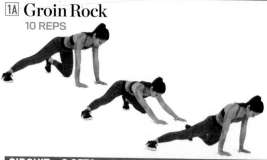

1B Bridge Hold
30 SECONDS

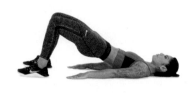

CIRCUIT > 3 SETS

2A Dumbbell Hip Thrust
10–12 REPS

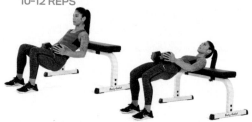

2B Goblet Sumo Squat
10–12 REPS

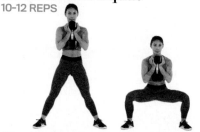

2C Tempo Dumbbell Romanian Deadlift
10–12 REPS

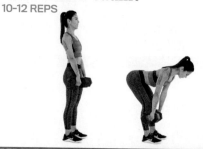

2D Alternating Lateral Goblet Squat
10–12 REPS

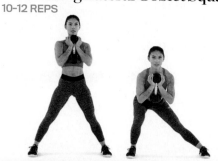

SUPERSET > 2 SETS

3A Plank with Alternating Rotation
10 REPS

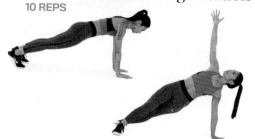

3B Bodyweight Split Squat
15 REPS

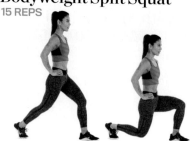

STAGE 1 > WORKOUT 4 > LOG

Use this space to record how much weight you use and how many reps you complete on each set. This will help you select the right weights and track your progress from week to week.

1A Groin Rock

WEEK	REPS	SET 1	SET 2
1	10		
2	10		
3	10		
4	10		

1B Bridge Hold

WEEK	REPS	SET 1	SET 2
1	30 seconds		
2	30 seconds		
3	30 seconds		
4	30 seconds		

2A Dumbbell Hip Thrust

WEEK	REPS	SET 1	SET 2	SET 3
1	10-12			
2	10-12			
3	10-12			
4	10-12			

2B Goblet Sumo Squat

WEEK	REPS	SET 1	SET 2	SET 3
1	10-12			
2	10-12			
3	10-12			
4	10-12			

2C Tempo Dumbbell Romanian Deadlift

WEEK	REPS	SET 1	SET 2	SET 3
1	10-12			
2	10-12			
3	10-12			
4	10-12			

2D Alternating Lateral Goblet Squat

WEEK	REPS	SET 1	SET 2	SET 3
1	10-12			
2	10-12			
3	10-12			
4	10-12			

3A Plank with Alternating Rotation

WEEK	REPS	SET 1	SET 2
1	10		
2	10		
3	10		
4	10		

3B Bodyweight Split Squat

WEEK	REPS	SET 1	SET 2
1	15		
2	15		
3	15		
4	15		

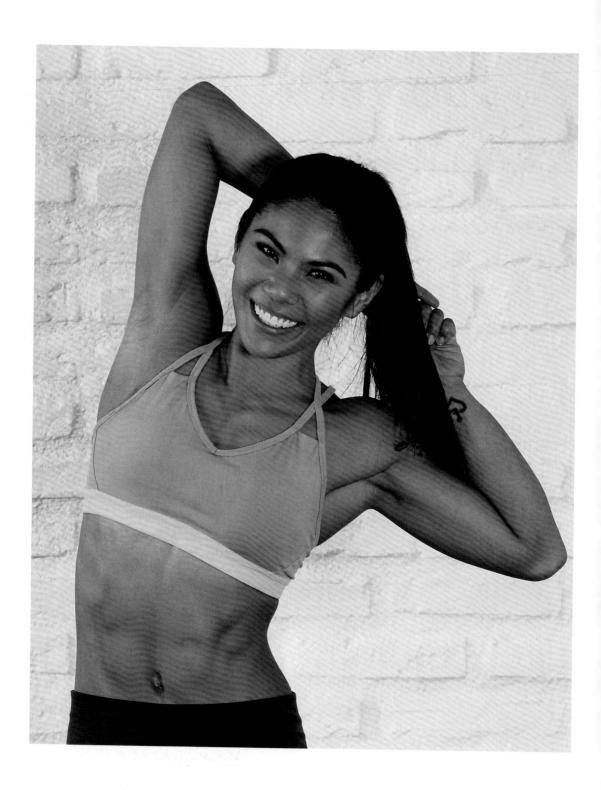

STAGE TWO

During Weeks 5 to 8, you'll start to incorporate bigger compound movements into the program to continually challenge your muscles and, by working your upper and lower body simultaneously, help you burn more calories and build more muscle with every rep. You'll also begin to bump up the weights you use while decreasing reps. This allows you to focus in on building strength. Lastly, working with a barbell will build the skills you need for workouts to come. All workouts take between 30 and 45 minutes.

STAGE 2 > WORKOUT 1

WARMUP > 2 SETS

1A Plank
30 SECONDS

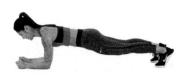

1B Side-Lying Shoulder Sweep
15 REPS

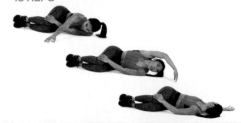

CIRCUIT > 4 SETS

2A Tempo Incline Pushup
10–12 REPS

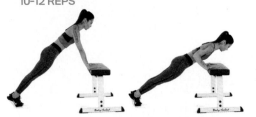

2B Dumbbell Bent-Over Row
10–12 REPS

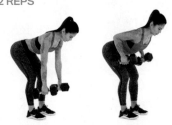

2C Seated Dumbbell Overhead Press
10–12 REPS

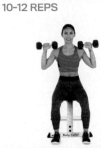
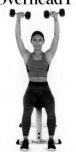

2D Kneeling Lat Pulldown
10–12 REPS

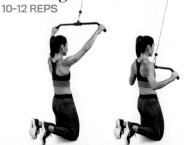

SUPERSET > 2 SETS

3A Suitcase Carry
20 REPS

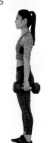
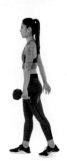

3B Seated Overhead Triceps Extension
10 REPS

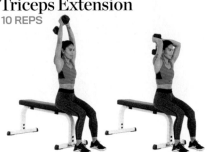

STAGE 2 > WORKOUT 1 > LOG

Use this space to record how much weight you use and how many reps you complete on each set. This will help you select the right weights and track your progress from week to week.

1A Plank

WEEK	REPS	SET 1	SET 2
5	30 seconds		
6	30 seconds		
7	30 seconds		
8	30 seconds		

1B Side-Lying Shoulder Sweep

WEEK	REPS	SET 1	SET 2
5	15		
6	15		
7	15		
8	15		

2A Tempo Incline Pushup

WEEK	REPS	SET 1	SET 2	SET 3	SET 4
5	10-12				
6	10-12				
7	10-12				
8	10-12				

2B Dumbbell Bent-Over Row

WEEK	REPS	SET 1	SET 2	SET 3	SET 4
5	10-12				
6	10-12				
7	10-12				
8	10-12				

2C Seated Dumbbell Overhead Press

WEEK	REPS	SET 1	SET 2	SET 3	SET 4
5	10-12				
6	10-12				
7	10-12				
8	10-12				

2D Kneeling Lat Pull-Down

WEEK	REPS	SET 1	SET 2	SET 3	SET 4
5	10-12				
6	10-12				
7	10-12				
8	10-12				

3A Suitcase Carry

WEEK	REPS	SET 1	SET 2
5	20		
6	20		
7	20		
8	20		

3B Seated Overhead Triceps Extension

WEEK	REPS	SET 1	SET 2
5	10		
6	10		
7	10		
8	10		

STAGE 2 > WORKOUT 2

WARMUP > 2 SETS

1A **Bridge Hold**
30 SECONDS

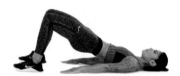

1B **Miniband Squat**
15 REPS

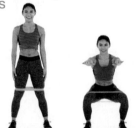

CIRCUIT > 4 SETS

2A **Goblet Squat**
10-12 REPS

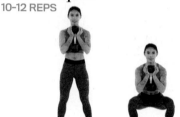

2B **Dumbbell Hip Thrust**
10-12 REPS

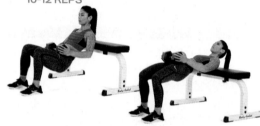

2C **Dumbbell Stepup**
10-12 REPS

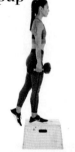

2D **Dumbbell Romanian Deadlift**
10-12 REPS

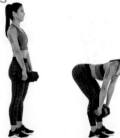

SUPERSET > 2 SETS

3A **Lateral Band Walk**
10 REPS

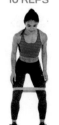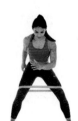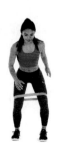

3B **Hollow-Body Hold**
30-60 SECONDS

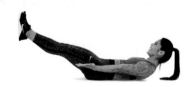

STAGE 2 > WORKOUT 2 > LOG

Use this space to record how much weight you use and how many reps you complete on each set. This will help you select the right weights and track your progress from week to week.

1A Bridge Hold

WEEK	REPS	SET 1	SET 2
5	30 seconds		
2	30 seconds		
3	30 seconds		
4	30 seconds		

1B Miniband Squat

WEEK	REPS	SET 1	SET 2
5	15		
2	15		
3	15		
4	15		

2A Goblet Squat

WEEK	REPS	SET 1	SET 2	SET 3	SET 4
5	10-12				
6	10-12				
7	10-12				
8	10-12				

2B Dumbbell Hip Thrust

WEEK	REPS	SET 1	SET 2	SET 3	SET 4
5	10-12				
6	10-12				
7	10-12				
8	10-12				

2C Dumbbell Stepup

WEEK	REPS	SET 1	SET 2	SET 3	SET 4
5	10-12				
6	10-12				
7	10-12				
8	10-12				

2D Dumbbell Romanian Deadlift

WEEK	REPS	SET 1	SET 2	SET 3	SET 4
5	10-12				
6	10-12				
7	10-12				
8	10-12				

3A Lateral Band Walk

WEEK	REPS	SET 1	SET 2
5	10		
2	10		
3	10		
4	10		

3B Hollow-Body Hold

WEEK	REPS	SET 1	SET 2
5	30-60 seconds		
2	30-60 seconds		
3	30-60 seconds		
4	30-60 seconds		

STAGE 2 > WORKOUT 3

WARMUP > 2 SETS

1A Side-Lying Shoulder Sweep
15 REPS

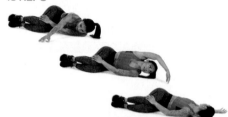

1B Alternating Plank Shoulder Tap
15 REPS

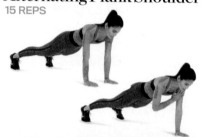

CIRCUIT > 4 SETS

2A Squat and Overhead Press
8–10 REPS

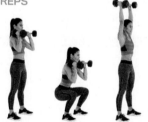

2B Alternating Plank Row
8–10 REPS

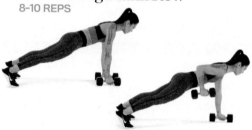

2C Incline Plyometric Pushup
8–10 REPS

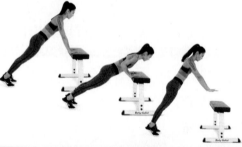

2D Alternating Reverse Lunge to Twist
8–10 REPS

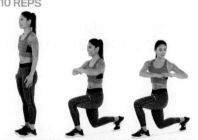

SUPERSET > 2 SETS

3A Wall-Sit Biceps Curl
10–12 REPS

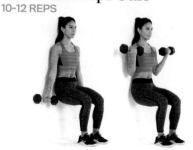

3B Alternating Lateral Bound
15 REPS

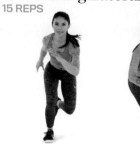

STAGE 2 > WORKOUT 3 > LOG

Use this space to record how much weight you use and how many reps you complete on each set. This will help you select the right weights and track your progress from week to week.

1A Side-Lying Shoulder Sweep

WEEK	REPS	SET 1	SET 2
5	15		
6	15		
7	15		
8	15		

1B Alternating Plank Shoulder Tap

WEEK	REPS	SET 1	SET 2
5	15		
6	15		
7	15		
8	15		

2A Squat and Overhead Press

WEEK	REPS	SET 1	SET 2	SET 3	SET 4
5	8-10				
6	8-10				
7	8-10				
8	8-10				

2B Alternating Plank Row

WEEK	REPS	SET 1	SET 2	SET 3	SET 4
5	8-10				
6	8-10				
7	8-10				
8	8-10				

2C Incline Plyometric Pushup

WEEK	REPS	SET 1	SET 2	SET 3	SET 4
5	8-10				
6	8-10				
7	8-10				
8	8-10				

2D Alternating Reverse Lunge to Twist

WEEK	REPS	SET 1	SET 2	SET 3	SET 4
5	8-10				
6	8-10				
7	8-10				
8	8-10				

3A Wall-Sit Biceps Curl

WEEK	REPS	SET 1	SET 2
5	10-12		
6	10-12		
7	10-12		
8	10-12		

3B Alternating Lateral Bound

WEEK	REPS	SET 1	SET 2
5	15		
6	15		
7	15		
8	15		

STAGE 2 > WORKOUT 4

WARMUP > 2 SETS

1A Prone Shoulder Squeeze
15 REPS

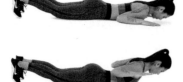

1B Miniband Squat
15 REPS

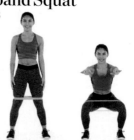

CIRCUIT > 4 SETS

2A Barbell Romanian Deadlift
8-10 REPS

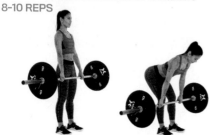

2B Barbell Bench Press
8-10 REPS

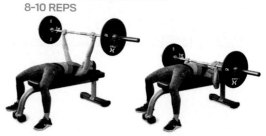

2C Barbell Front Squat
8-10 REPS

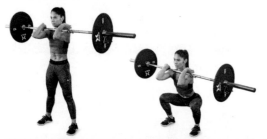

2D Barbell Bent-Over Row
8-10 REPS

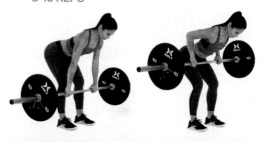

SUPERSET > 2 SETS

3A Band-Assisted Chinup
MAX

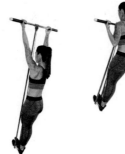

3B Windshield Wiper
10 REPS

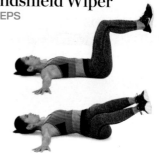

STAGE 2 > WORKOUT 4 > LOG

Use this space to record how much weight you use and how many reps you complete on each set. This will help you select the right weights and track your progress from week to week.

1A Prone Shoulder Squeeze

WEEK	REPS	SET 1	SET 2
5	15		
6	15		
7	15		
8	15		

1B Miniband Squat

WEEK	REPS	SET 1	SET 2
5	15		
6	15		
7	15		
8	15		

2A Barbell Romanian Deadlift

WEEK	REPS	SET 1	SET 2	SET 3	SET 4
5	8-10				
6	8-10				
7	8-10				
8	8-10				

2B Barbell Bench Press

WEEK	REPS	SET 1	SET 2	SET 3	SET 4
5	8-10				
6	8-10				
7	8-10				
8	8-10				

2C Barbell Front Squat

WEEK	REPS	SET 1	SET 2	SET 3	SET 4
5	8-10				
6	8-10				
7	8-10				
8	8-10				

2D Barbell Bent-Over Row

WEEK	REPS	SET 1	SET 2	SET 3	SET 4
5	8-10				
6	8-10				
7	8-10				
8	8-10				

3A Band-Assisted Chinup

WEEK	REPS	SET 1	SET 2
5	Max		
6	Max		
7	Max		
8	Max		

3B Windshield Wiper

WEEK	REPS	SET 1	SET 2
5	10		
6	10		
7	10		
8	10		

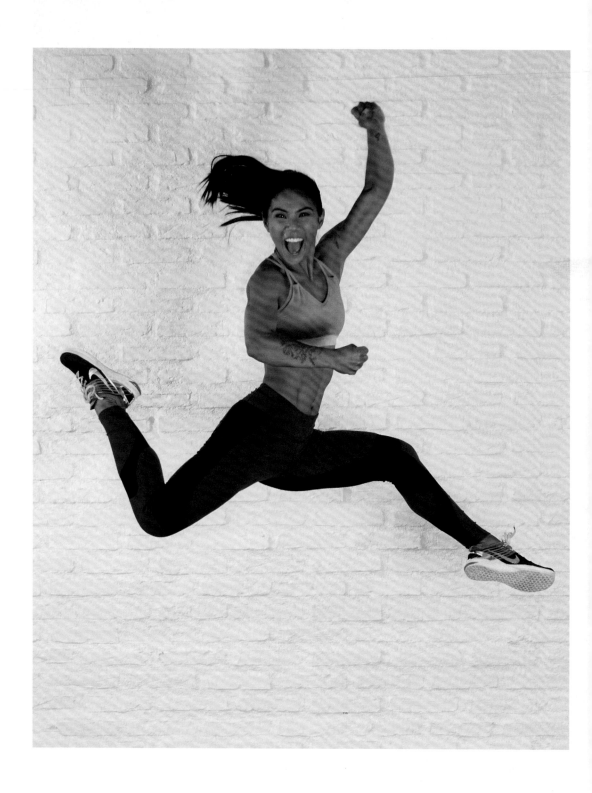

STAGE THREE

In Weeks 9 to 12, you'll decrease the number of reps you complete when performing barbell work so that you can lift really heavy! This is when big changes happen in both your body and mind. So get ready to feel like a badass, and don't be afraid to push yourself. During this stage, you'll also work on building muscular endurance so that you'll be able to not only generate a high level of force, but also do so for extended periods of time. All workouts take between 30 and 45 minutes.

STAGE 3 > WORKOUT 1

WARMUP > 2 SETS

1A Bird Dog
10 REPS

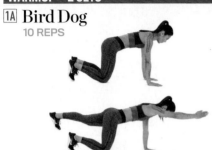

1B Prone Shoulder Squeeze
15 REPS

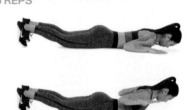

CIRCUIT > 4 SETS

2A Squat and Overhead Press
8-10 REPS

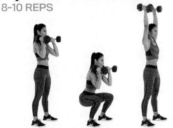

2B Inverted Row
8-10 REPS

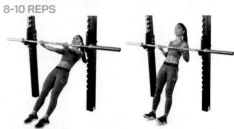

2C Half-Kneeling Low-to-High Dumbbell Chop
8-10 REPS

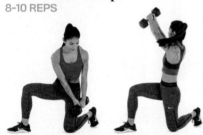

2D Alternating Dumbbell Lateral Lunge
8-10 REPS

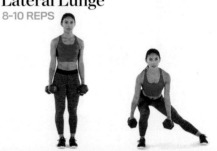

SUPERSET > 2 SETS

3A Suitcase Carry
20 REPS

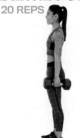
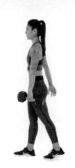

3B Plank Elevator
10 REPS

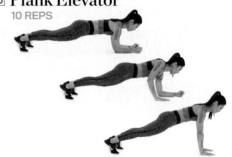

STAGE 3 > WORKOUT 1 > LOG

Use this space to record how much weight you use and how many reps you complete on each set. This will help you select the right weights and track your progress from week to week.

1A Bird Dog

WEEK	REPS	SET 1	SET 2
9	10		
10	10		
11	10		
12	10		

1B Prone Shoulder Squeeze

WEEK	REPS	SET 1	SET 2
9	15		
10	15		
11	15		
12	15		

2A Squat and Overhead Press

WEEK	REPS	SET 1	SET 2	SET 3	SET 4
9	8-10				
10	8-10				
11	8-10				
12	8-10				

2B Inverted Row

WEEK	REPS	SET 1	SET 2	SET 3	SET 4
9	8-10				
10	8-10				
11	8-10				
12	8-10				

2C Half-Kneeling Low-to-High Dumbbell Chop

WEEK	REPS	SET 1	SET 2	SET 3	SET 4
9	8-10				
10	8-10				
11	8-10				
12	8-10				

2D Alternating Dumbbell Lateral Lunge

WEEK	REPS	SET 1	SET 2	SET 3	SET 4
9	8-10				
10	8-10				
11	8-10				
12	8-10				

3A Suitcase Carry

WEEK	REPS	SET 1	SET 2
9	20		
10	20		
11	20		
12	20		

3B Plank Elevator

WEEK	REPS	SET 1	SET 2
9	10		
10	10		
11	10		
12	10		

STAGE 3 > WORKOUT 2

WARMUP > 2 SETS

1A Side-Lying Shoulder Sweep
15 REPS

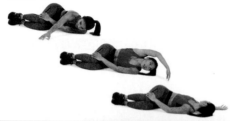

1B Groin Rock
10 REPS

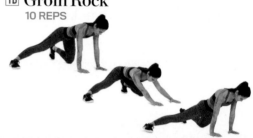

CIRCUIT > 4 SETS

2A Dumbbell Single-Leg Romanian Deadlift
8-10 REPS

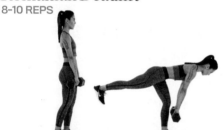

2B Plank Row Rotation and Extension
8-10 REPS

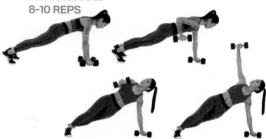

2C Dumbbell Sumo Deadlift
8-10 REPS

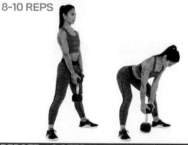

2D Half-Kneeling High-to-Low Cable Chop
8-10 REPS

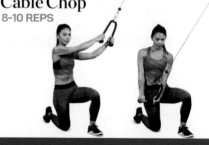

SUPERSET > 2 SETS

3A Side Plank
20-60 SECONDS

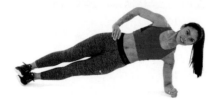

3B Miniband Side-Lying Hip Abduction
10 REPS

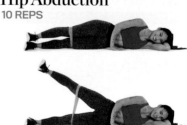

STAGE 3 > WORKOUT 2 > LOG

Use this space to record how much weight you use and how many reps you complete on each set. This will help you select the right weights and track your progress from week to week.

1A Side-Lying Shoulder Sweep

WEEK	REPS	SET 1	SET 2
9	15		
10	15		
11	15		
12	15		

1B Groin Rock

WEEK	REPS	SET 1	SET 2
9	10		
10	10		
11	10		
12	10		

2A Dumbbell Single-Leg Romanian Deadlift

WEEK	REPS	SET 1	SET 2	SET 3	SET 4
9	8-10				
10	8-10				
11	8-10				
12	8-10				

2B Plank Row Rotation and Extension

WEEK	REPS	SET 1	SET 2	SET 3	SET 4
9	8-10				
10	8-10				
11	8-10				
12	8-10				

2C Dumbbell Sumo Deadlift

WEEK	REPS	SET 1	SET 2	SET 3	SET 4
9	8-10				
10	8-10				
11	8-10				
12	8-10				

2D Half-Kneeling High-to-Low Cable Chop

WEEK	REPS	SET 1	SET 2	SET 3	SET 4
9	8-10				
10	8-10				
11	8-10				
12	8-10				

3A Side Plank

WEEK	REPS	SET 1	SET 2
9	20-60 seconds		
10	20-60 seconds		
11	20-60 seconds		
12	20-60 seconds		

3B Miniband Side-Lying Hip Abduction

WEEK	REPS	SET 1	SET 2
9	10		
10	10		
11	10		
12	10		

STAGE 3 > WORKOUT 3

WARMUP > 2 SETS

1A Dead Bug
10 REPS

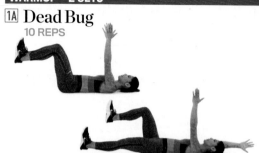

1B Prone Shoulder Squeeze
15 REPS

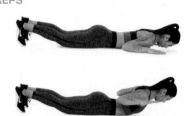

CIRCUIT > 4 SETS

2A Barbell Front Squat
6–8 REPS

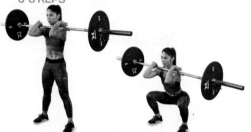

2B Barbell Bent-Over Row
6–8 REPS

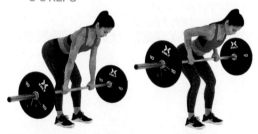

2C Barbell Reverse Lunge
6–8 REPS

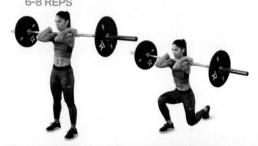

2D Band-Assisted Chinup
6–8 REPS

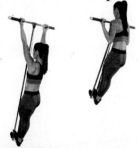

SUPERSET > 2 SETS

3A Plank with Alternating Hip Dip
10 REPS

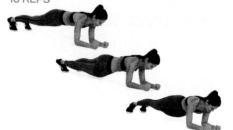

3B Rack-Position Carry
30 REPS

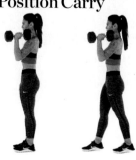

STAGE 3 > WORKOUT 3 > LOG

Use this space to record how much weight you use and how many reps you complete on each set. This will help you select the right weights and track your progress from week to week.

1A Dead Bug

WEEK	REPS	SET 1	SET 2
9	10		
10	10		
11	10		
12	10		

1B Prone Shoulder Squeeze

WEEK	REPS	SET 1	SET 2
9	15		
10	15		
11	15		
12	15		

2A Barbell Front Squat

WEEK	REPS	SET 1	SET 2	SET 3	SET 4
9	6-8				
10	6-8				
11	6-8				
12	6-8				

2B Barbell Bent-Over Row

WEEK	REPS	SET 1	SET 2	SET 3	SET 4
9	6-8				
10	6-8				
11	6-8				
12	6-8				

2C Barbell Reverse Lunge

WEEK	REPS	SET 1	SET 2	SET 3	SET 4
9	6-8				
10	6-8				
11	6-8				
12	6-8				

2D Band-Assisted Chinup

WEEK	REPS	SET 1	SET 2	SET 3	SET 4
9	6-8				
10	6-8				
11	6-8				
12	6-8				

3A Plank with Alternating Hip Dip

WEEK	REPS	SET 1	SET 2
9	10		
10	10		
11	10		
12	10		

3B Rack-Position Carry

WEEK	REPS	SET 1	SET 2
9	30		
10	30		
11	30		
12	30		

STAGE 3 > WORKOUT 4

WARMUP > 2 SETS

1A Glute Bridge
15 REPS

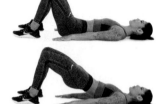

1B Side-Lying Shoulder Sweep
15 REPS

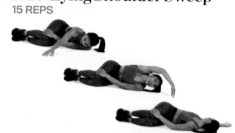

CIRCUIT > 4 SETS

2A Barbell Romanian Deadlift
6–8 REPS

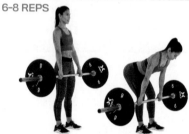

2B Barbell Bench Press
6–8 REPS

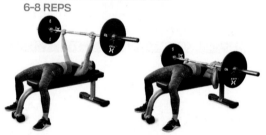

2C Barbell Hip Thrust
6–8 REPS

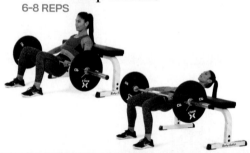

2D Barbell Overhead Press
6–8 REPS

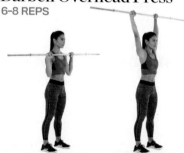

SUPERSET > 2 SETS

3A Superman
15 REPS

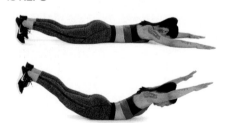

3B Windshield Wiper
10 REPS

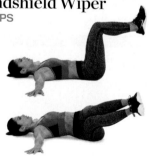

STAGE 3 > WORKOUT 4 > LOG

Use this space to record how much weight you use and how many reps you complete on each set. This will help you select the right weights and track your progress from week to week.

1A Glute Bridge

WEEK	REPS	SET 1	SET 2
9	15		
10	15		
11	15		
12	15		

1B Side-Lying Shoulder Sweep

WEEK	REPS	SET 1	SET 2
9	15		
10	15		
11	15		
12	15		

2A Barbell Romanian Deadlift

WEEK	REPS	SET 1	SET 2	SET 3	SET 4
9	6-8				
10	6-8				
11	6-8				
12	6-8				

2B Barbell Bench Press

WEEK	REPS	SET 1	SET 2	SET 3
9	6-8			
10	6-8			
11	6-8			
12	6-8			

2C Barbell Hip Thrust

WEEK	REPS	SET 1	SET 2	SET 3	SET 4
9	6-8				
10	6-8				
11	6-8				
12	6-8				

2D Barbell Overhead Press

WEEK	REPS	SET 1	SET 2	SET 3	SET 4
9	6-8				
10	6-8				
11	6-8				
12	6-8				

3A Superman

WEEK	REPS	SET 1	SET 2
9	15		
10	15		
11	15		
12	15		

3B Windshield Wiper

WEEK	REPS	SET 1	SET 2
9	10		
10	10		
11	10		
12	10		

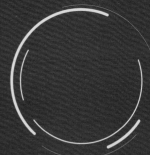

THE EXERCISE GUIDE

Here, you can find directions on how to do every exercise in the program, including variations you can perform to make the moves more or less difficult, work around cranky knees or wrists, and get the most out of every rep. See the next page for an index that will help you locate each move.

MOBILITY & ACTIVATION EXERCISES

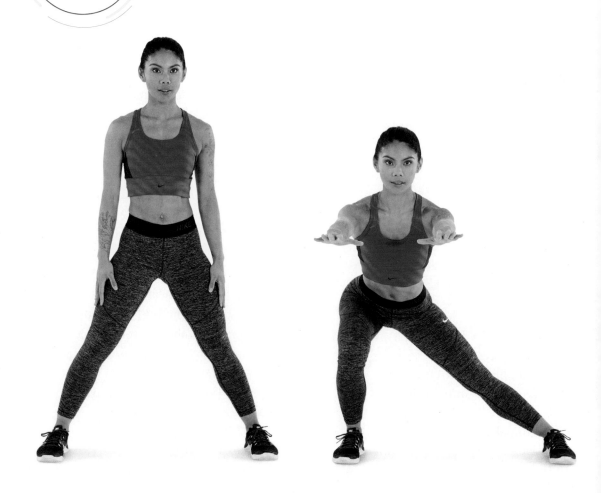

Alternating Lateral Squat

Stand tall with your feet twice shoulder-width apart. From here, shift your weight to your right leg and push your hips back and bend your right knee to lower as far as you can while keeping your left leg straight. Pause, then press through your right heel to return to start. Repeat on the opposite side. That's one rep.

MOBILITY & ACTIVATION EXERCISES

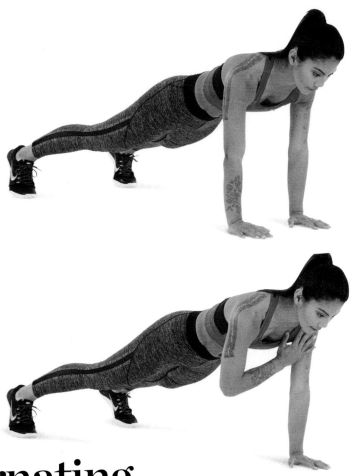

Alternating Plank Shoulder Tap

Assume a pushup position. Your body should form a straight line from your head to your heels. Brace your core and pull your shoulders back away from your ears. Pretend you're digging your hands into the floor and pulling them toward your feet. This is your starting position. Slowly and under control, lift your right hand off the floor and touch your left shoulder. Pause, then lower your hand to return to the starting position. Repeat on the opposite side. That's one rep.

MOBILITY & ACTIVATION EXERCISES

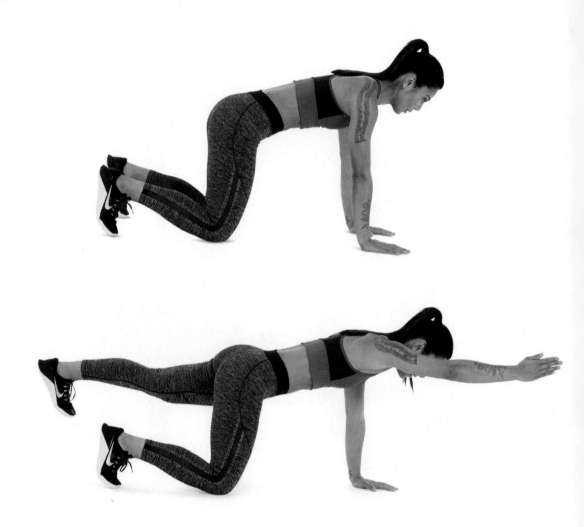

Bird Dog

Get down on your hands and knees with your palms flat on the floor and shoulder-width apart. Hold your back flat and brace your core. From here, raise your right arm and left leg until they're parallel to the floor, keeping your torso stationary as you do so. Pause, then slowly lower your arm and leg to return to start. Repeat on the opposite side. That's one rep.

MOBILITY & ACTIVATION EXERCISES

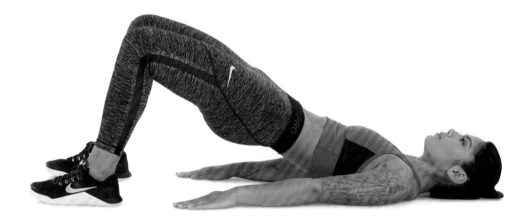

Bridge Hold

Lie faceup on the floor with your knees bent and feet flat on the floor, hip-width apart and about 6 to 8 inches from your glutes. Brace your core. From here, push through your heels and squeeze your glutes to lift your hips so that your body forms a straight line from shoulders to knees, and your shins are vertical. Hold for the prescribed time.

MOBILITY & ACTIVATION EXERCISES

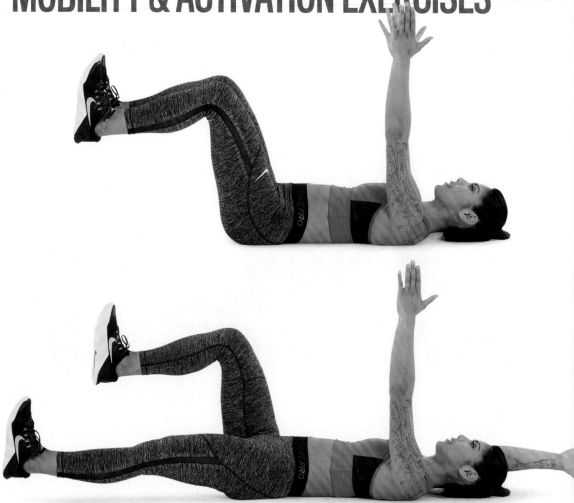

Dead Bug

Lie faceup on the floor with your arms and legs lifted toward the ceiling, knees bent. Press your lower back into the floor and brace your core. While maintaining this flat-back position, lower your right arm toward the floor above your head and your left leg toward the floor, straightening your knee as you do so. Pause when both are nearly parallel to the floor. Squeeze your abs to pull your arm and leg back to start. Repeat on the opposite side. That's one rep.

(WANT AN EXTRA CORE CHALLENGE?)

Keep your legs straight throughout the entire exercise.

MOBILITY & ACTIVATION EXERCISES

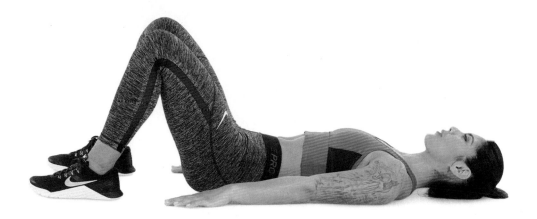

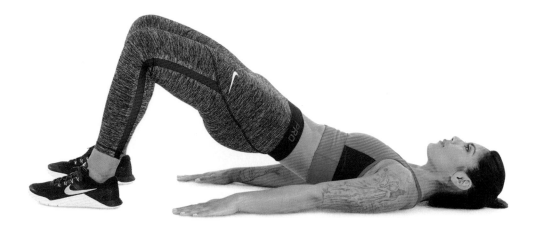

Glute Bridge

Lie faceup on the floor with your knees bent and feet flat on the floor, hip-width apart and about 6 to 8 inches from your glutes. Brace your core. From here, push through your heels and squeeze your glutes to lift your hips until your body forms a straight line from shoulders to knees, and your shins are vertical. Pause, then slowly lower your hips to return to start. That's one rep.

MOBILITY & ACTIVATION EXERCISES

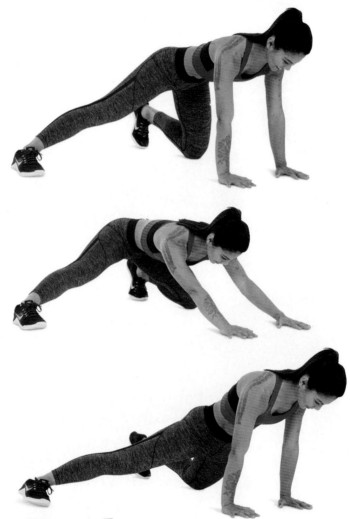

Groin Rock

Get on your hands and knees with your hands directly under your shoulders and knees under your hips. Extend your right leg out to the side so that your leg is perpendicular to your body and your right foot is flat on the floor. This is your starting position. Shift your glutes back toward your left heel, then shift your weight forward so that your shoulders move past your wrists, and drive your hips to the floor. Return to the starting position. That's one rep. Complete all reps, then repeat on opposite side.

MOBILITY & ACTIVATION EXERCISES

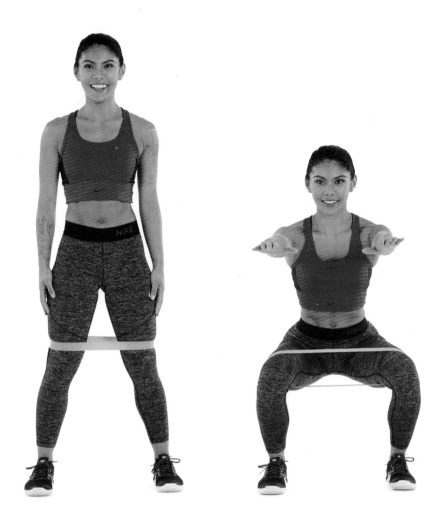

Miniband Squat

Loop a miniband around both legs, just above your knees, and stand tall with your feet shoulder-width apart. Brace your core. From here, push your hips back and bend your knees to lower your body as far as you can, pressing outward against the band with your knees. Pause, then push through your heels to return to start. That's one rep.

MOBILITY & ACTIVATION EXERCISES

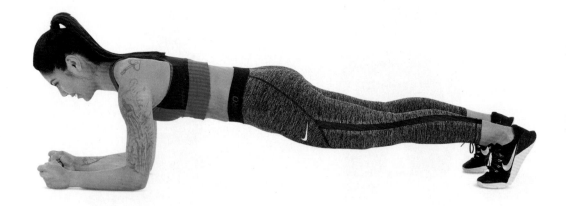

Plank

Assume a pushup position, but rest your weight on your forearms instead of on your hands. Your elbows should be under your shoulders. Your body should form a straight line from your head to your heels. Brace your core and pull your shoulders back away from your ears. Pretend you're digging your forearms into the floor and pulling them toward your feet. Hold for the prescribed time.

MOBILITY & ACTIVATION EXERCISES

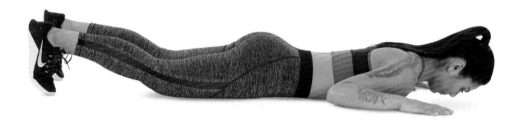

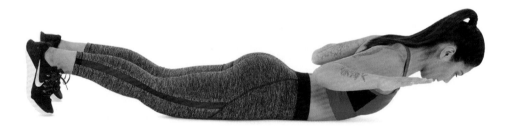

Prone Shoulder Squeeze

Lie facedown on the floor with your arms flat on the floor, elbows bent and hands palms-down. From here, pinch your shoulder blades back and together and raise your hands and elbows off the floor. Hold for 2 seconds, then relax your arms and shoulder blades to return to start. That's one rep.

MOBILITY & ACTIVATION EXERCISES

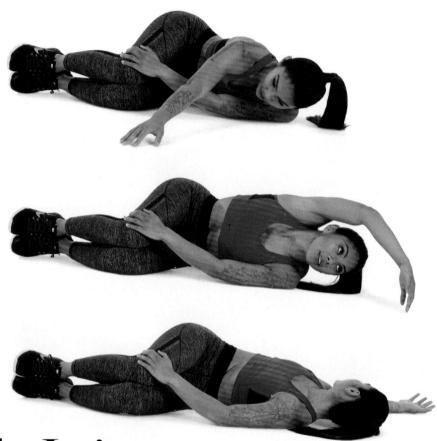

Side-Lying Shoulder Sweep

Lie on your left side in a fetal position, hips and knees bent 90 degrees. Your knees should be stacked. Place your left hand on your top knee, and brace your core. Reach your right hand in front of you on the floor. From here, sweep your right hand up and around your body in a half circle to reach behind you as far as you can without letting your knees un-stack or raise off of the floor. Hold for 3 to 5 seconds, then reverse the motion to return to start. That's one rep. Complete all reps, then repeat on the opposite side.

Hollow-Body Hold

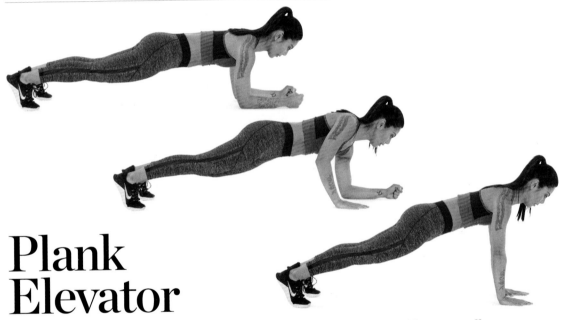

Lie faceup on the floor with your legs extended toward the ceiling so they are perpendicular to the floor. Squeeze your abs to raise your head and shoulders just off the floor while simultaneously lowering your legs as close to the floor as possible while keeping your lower back against the floor. Hold for the prescribed time.

Plank Elevator

Assume a pushup position, but place your forearms on the floor so that your elbows are under your shoulders. Brace your core and pull your shoulders back. Pretend you're digging your forearms into the floor and pulling them toward your feet. This is your starting position. Lift your right forearm and place your right hand on the floor. In one movement, straighten your right arm as you simultaneously place your left hand on the floor and straighten your left arm. Reverse the movement by placing your right forearm on the floor and then your left. That's one rep. Repeat, this time starting with your left hand.

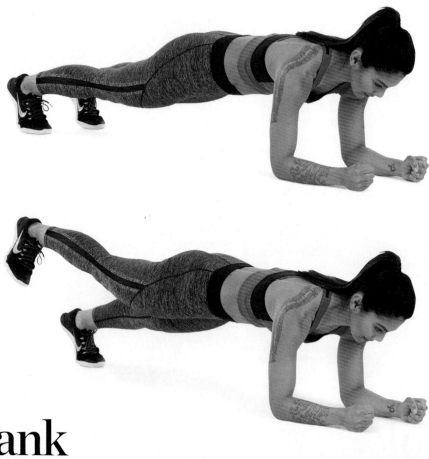

Plank
with Alternating Leg Lift

Assume a pushup position, but place your forearms on the floor so that your elbows are under your shoulders. Your body should form a straight line from head to heels. Brace your core and pull your shoulders back away from your ears. Pretend you're digging your forearms into the floor and pulling them toward your feet. This is your starting position. Raise your right foot from the floor, keeping your torso stationary as you do so. Pause, then lower your foot to the floor to return to the starting position. Repeat on the opposite side. That's one rep.

CORE EXERCISES > STABILITY

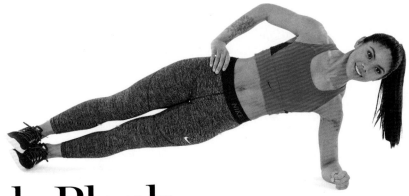

Side Plank

Lie on the floor on your left side with your legs straight and feet stacked. Prop your upper body up on your left forearm with your elbow bent and directly underneath your shoulder. Your body should form a straight line from head to heels. Rest your right hand on your hip. Hold for the prescribed time, then repeat on the opposite site.

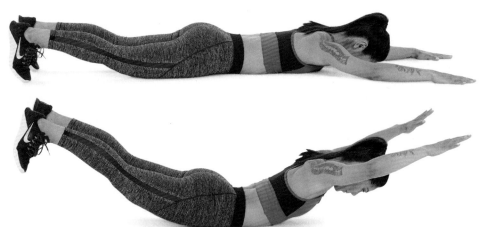

Superman

Lie on the floor on your stomach with your arms out straight over your head. Brace your core. From here, squeeze your back, shoulders, and glutes to raise your arms and legs just off of the floor. Pause, then slowly release the tension to lower your arms and legs back to start. That's one rep.

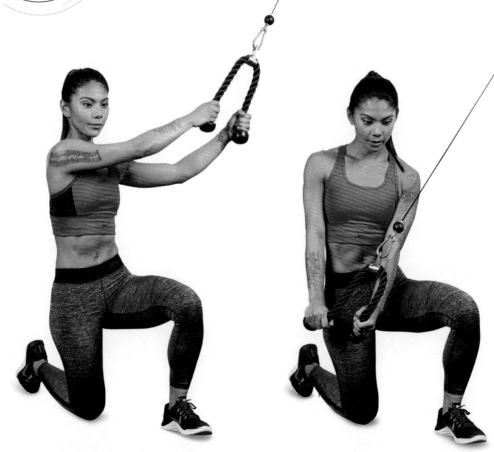

Half-Kneeling High-to-Low Cable Chop

In front of a cable machine with a rope or stirrup handle attached, get into a half-kneeling position with your right knee down. Grab the handle above your left shoulder, your arms straight. Brace your core. This is your starting position. Rotate your torso and pull the handle down and to the right. Reverse the movement to return to the starting position. That's one rep. Complete all reps, then repeat on the opposite side.

CORE EXERCISES > ROTATIONS

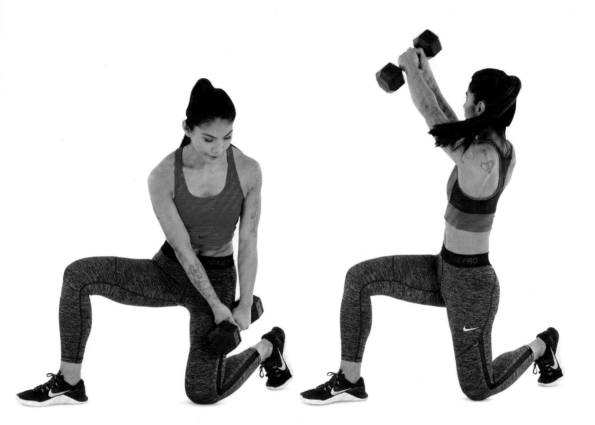

Half-Kneeling Low-to-High Dumbbell Chop

Get into a half-kneeling position with your left knee down. Rotate to the left and bend at your hips to hold a dumbbell with both hands just outside of your left thigh, arms straight. Brace your core. This is your starting position. From here, lift the dumbbell diagonally up and across your body until it is above your right shoulder. Slowly reverse the movement to return to the starting position. That's one rep. Complete all reps and then repeat on the opposite side.

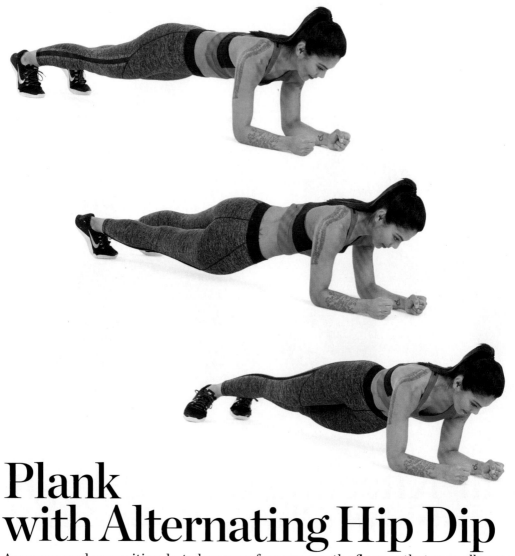

Plank
with Alternating Hip Dip

Assume a pushup position, but place your forearms on the floor so that your elbows are under your shoulders. Your body should form a straight line from head to heels. Brace your core and pull your shoulders back away from your ears. Pretend you're digging your forearms into the floor and pulling them toward your feet. This is your starting position. From here, lower your right hip until it almost touches the floor. Pause, then raise your hip to return to the starting position. Repeat on the opposite side. That's one rep.

CORE EXERCISES > ROTATIONS

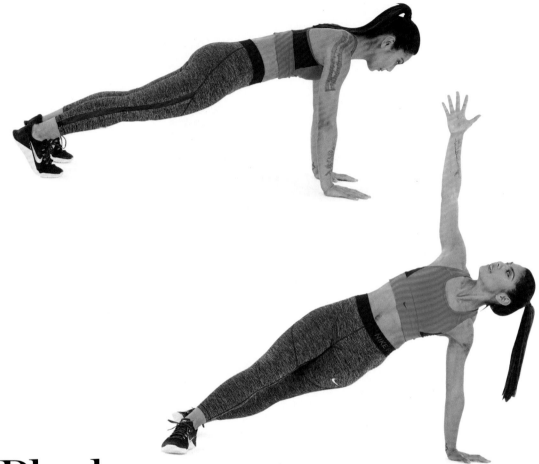

Plank
with Alternating Rotation

Assume a pushup position. Your body should form a straight line from your head to your heels. Brace your core and pull your shoulders back away from your ears. Pretend you're digging your hands into the floor and pulling them toward your feet. This is your starting position. From here, lift your right hand, rotate your hips, and swivel your feet to get into a side plank, extending your right arm straight toward the ceiling. Pause, then reverse the movement to return to the starting position. Repeat on the opposite side. That's one rep.

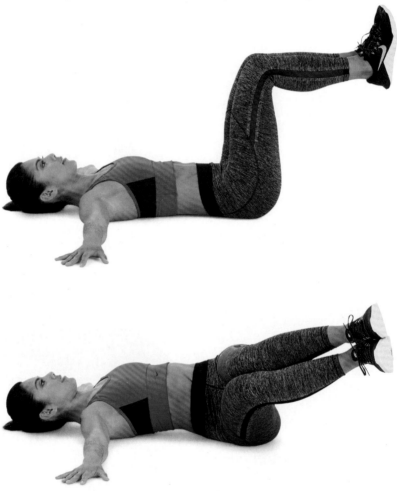

Windshield Wiper

Lie faceup on the floor with your arms straight out from your sides, palms facing down. Raise your feet off the floor so that your knees and hips are both bent to 90 degrees. This is your starting position. Brace your core and, keeping your legs together, lower them to the right as far as you can without lifting your shoulders off the floor. Pause, then reverse the movement to return to the starting position. Repeat on the opposite side. That's one rep.

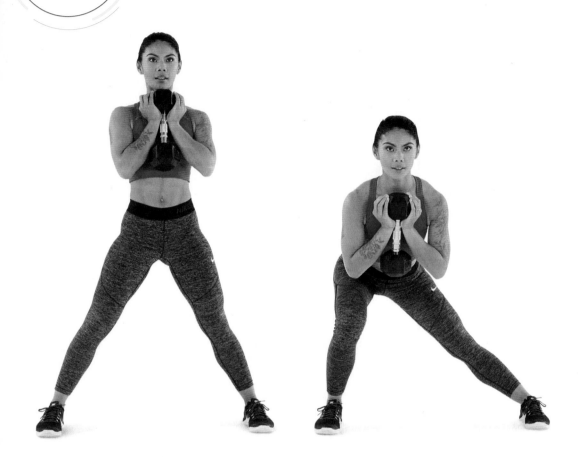

Alternating Lateral Goblet Squat

Hold a dumbbell vertically in front of your chest, with both hands cupping the top end of the weight. Stand tall with your feet twice shoulder-width apart. From here, shift your weight to your right leg, push your hips back, and bend your right knee to lower your body as far as you can while keeping your left leg straight. Pause, then press through your right heel to return to start. Repeat on the opposite side. That's one rep.

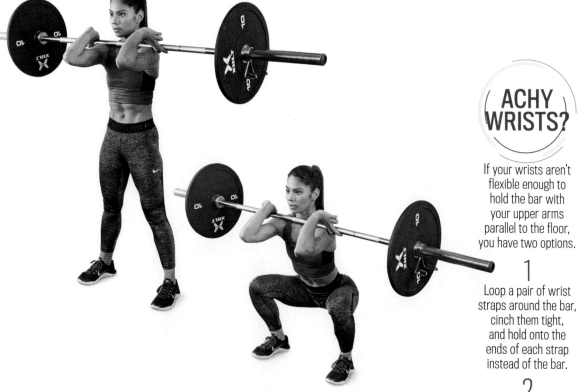

ACHY WRISTS?

If your wrists aren't flexible enough to hold the bar with your upper arms parallel to the floor, you have two options.

1

Loop a pair of wrist straps around the bar, cinch them tight, and hold onto the ends of each strap instead of the bar.

2

Hold the barbell in a crossed-arm position: With your arms out straight in front of you, position the bar against the front of your shoulders. Then, keeping your upper arms parallel to the floor, bend both elbows and cross your forearms and hold the bar in place against your shoulders with your hands.

Barbell Front Squat

Stand facing a barbell that's positioned on a squat rack just lower than shoulder height. Grasp the bar with an overhand grip, dip your knees, and let the bar roll back to the tips of your fingers until it rests securely on the front of your shoulders. Raise your upper arms until they're parallel to the floor. (The bar will stay in place as long as you don't allow your elbows to drop as you squat.) Take a step back and set your feet shoulder-width apart. This is your starting position. Keeping your torso as upright as you can, push your hips back, bend your knees, and lower your body until your thighs are at least parallel to the floor. Press your body up to return to the starting position. That's one rep.

LOWER-BODY EXERCISES > SQUATS

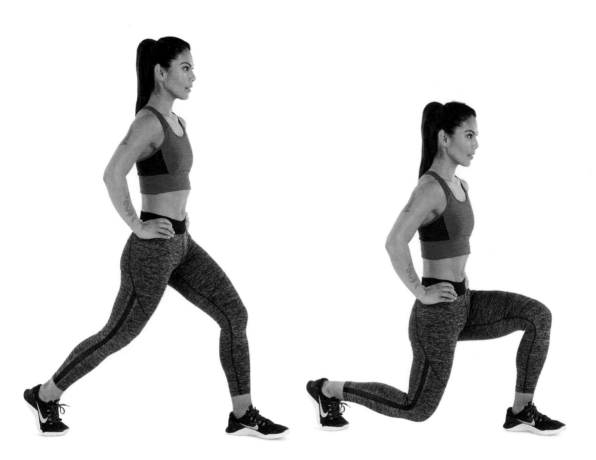

Bodyweight Split Squat

Stand tall in a staggered stance with your feet hip-width apart and your hands on your hips. Pull your shoulders back and brace your core. From here, bend your knees to lower your body toward the floor. Pause, then press through your front foot to return to start. That's one rep. Complete all reps and then repeat on the opposite side.

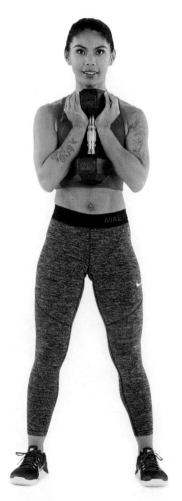

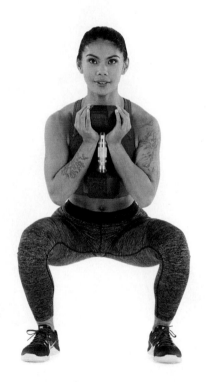

Goblet Squat

Hold a dumbbell vertically in front of your chest, with both hands cupping the top end of the weight. Stand tall with your feet just greater than shoulder-width apart. Brace your core. This is your starting position. From here, push your hips back and bend your knees to lower your body until your thighs are parallel to the floor (or as low as you can comfortably go). Pause, then push through your heels to return to the starting position. That's one rep.

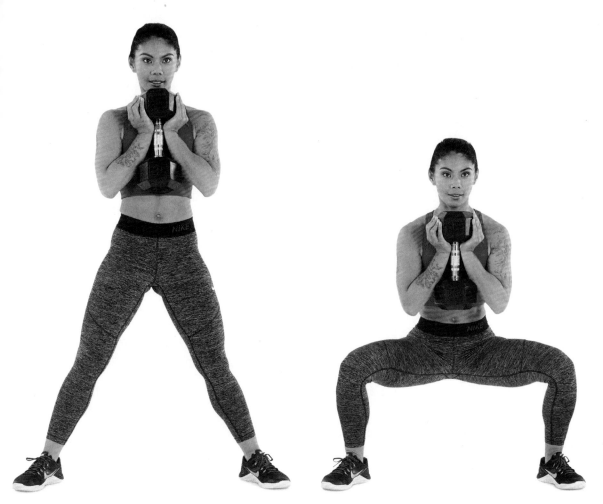

Goblet Sumo Squat

Hold a dumbbell vertically in front of your chest, with both hands cupping the top end of the weight. Stand tall with your feet twice shoulder-width apart, toes pointed diagonally away from your body. Brace your core. This is your starting position. Push your hips back and bend your knees to lower your body until your thighs are parallel to the floor (or as low as you can comfortably go). Pause, then push through your heels to return to the starting position. That's one rep.

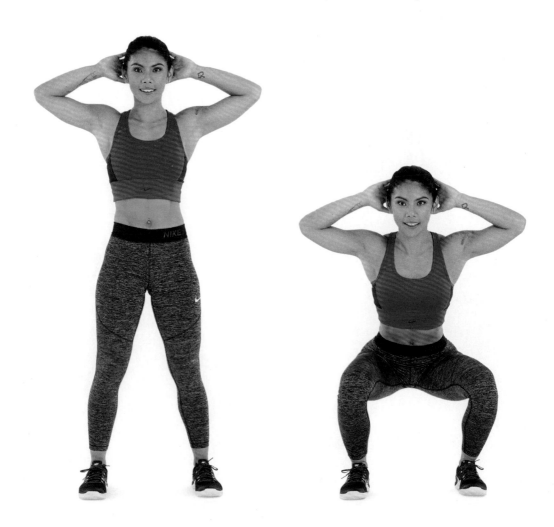

Prisoner Squat

Stand tall with your feet slightly wider than shoulder-width apart and your hands behind your head. Pull your elbows and shoulders back, and brace your core. From here, push your hips back and bend your knees to lower your body as far as you can. Pause, then push through your heels to return to start. That's one rep.

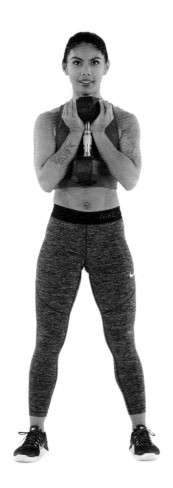
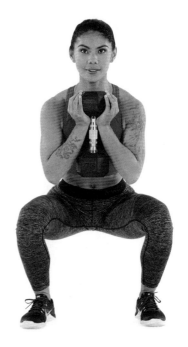

Tempo Goblet Squat

Hold a dumbbell vertically in front of your chest, with both hands cupping the top end of the weight. Stand tall with your feet just greater than shoulder-width apart. Brace your core. This is your starting position. From here, slowly push your hips back and bend your knees to lower your body until your thighs are parallel to the floor (or as low as you can comfortably go), taking four seconds to do so. Pause for one second, then push through your heels to return to start in one second. That's one rep.

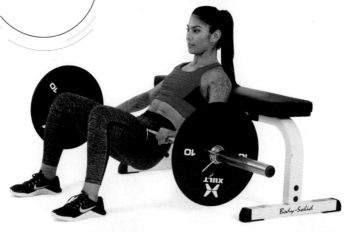

This can be a cumbersome move to set up. Make it simple by using a fixed bench that won't scoot around (consider commandeering the cable row station's bench), and your gym's rubber bumper plates. Place the loaded barbell on the floor, and the barbell will rest high enough off of the floor that you can slip your hips under the bar to get into the starting position.

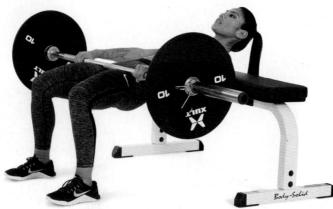

(OUCH!

Barbell Hip Thrust

Place a loaded barbell on the floor a few feet in front of a flat bench. Sit on the floor with your back pressed up against the long side of the bench and your legs out in front of you, under the barbell. Roll the barbell toward you until it is across the top of your hips, bend your knees, and place your feet flat on the floor about 6 to 8 inches from your glutes. Brace your core and lift your hips so that your butt is hovering off the floor. This is your starting position. Push through your heels and squeeze your glutes to raise your hips until your body forms a straight line from shoulders to knees, and your shins are vertical. Pause, then slowly lower your hips to return to your starting position. That's one rep.

If the weight of the barbell hurts the top of your hips, ask the staff at your gym if they have a hip pad that you can use. A rectangular piece of foam, it sits directly between your hips and the weight to keep you comfy and bruise-free.

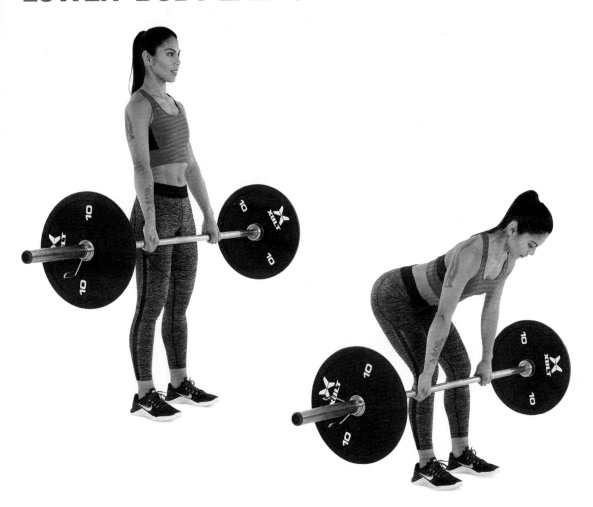

Barbell Romanian Deadlift

Stand tall with your feet hip-width apart and hold a barbell against your thighs with an overhand grip that's just wider than shoulder-width apart. Pull your shoulder blades together and brace your core. From here, bend at your hips to lower your torso until it is almost parallel to the floor (or you feel a stretch in your hamstrings). Drive through your heels and squeeze your glutes to thrust your hips forward and return to a standing position. That's one rep.

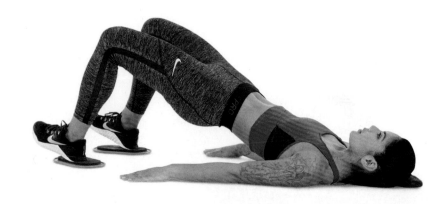

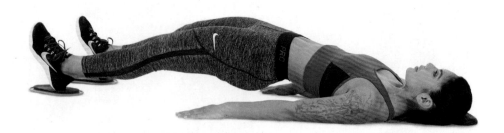

Bodyweight Hamstring Curl

Lie faceup on the floor with your knees bent and your heels on top of sliders or a towel on the floor, hip-width apart and about 12 inches from your glutes. Brace your core, push through your heels, and squeeze your glutes to lift your hips so that your body forms a straight line from shoulders to knees. This is your starting position. From here, slide your heels out to straighten your legs. Pause, then slide your heels back to your glutes to return to the starting position. That's one rep.

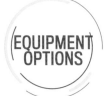

EQUIPMENT OPTIONS

Towels are great for performing this move at home on any hard floors. But you can also perform it with your feet on top of Valslides or even a stability ball.

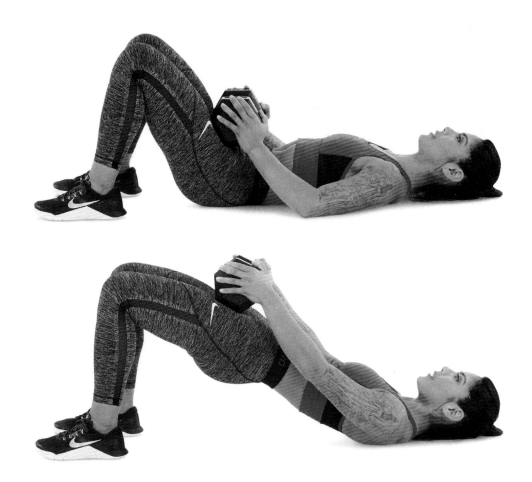

Dumbbell Glute Bridge

Lie faceup on the floor with your knees bent and feet flat on the floor, hip-width apart and about 6 to 8 inches from your glutes. Hold a dumbbell by both ends across the top of your hips, and brace your core. From here, push through your heels and squeeze your glutes to raise your hips until your body forms a straight line from shoulders to knees, and your shins are vertical. Pause, then lower your hips to return to start. That's one rep.

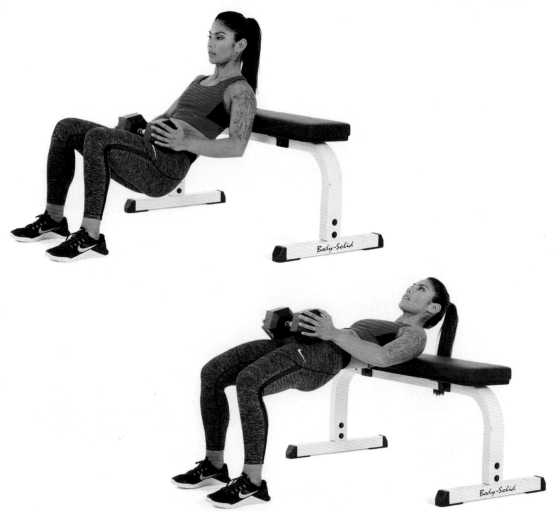

Dumbbell Hip Thrust

Sit with your back pressed up against the long side of a flat bench and your feet flat on the floor about 6 to 8 inches from your glutes. Hold a dumbbell by both ends across the top of your hips. Brace your core and lift your hips so that your butt is hovering off the floor. This is your starting position. From here, push through your heels and squeeze your glutes to lift your hips until your body forms a straight line from shoulders to knees, and your shins are vertical. Pause, then lower your hips to return to the starting position. That's one rep.

LOWER-BODY EXERCISES > HIP HINGES

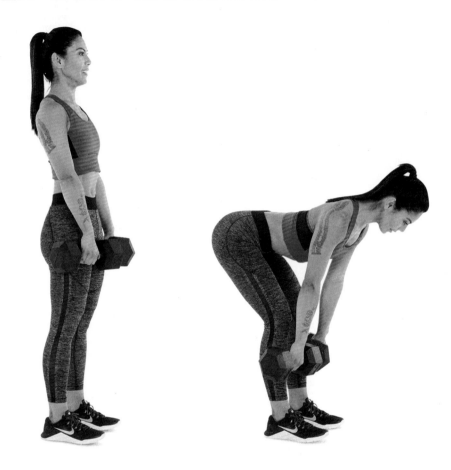

Dumbbell Romanian Deadlift

Stand tall with your feet hip-width apart and hold a dumbbell in each hand with an overhand grip in front of your hips. Pull your shoulder blades together and brace your core. From here, bend at your hips to lower your torso until it is almost parallel to the floor (or you feel a stretch in your hamstrings). Drive through your heels and squeeze your glutes to thrust your hips forward and return to a standing position. That's one rep.

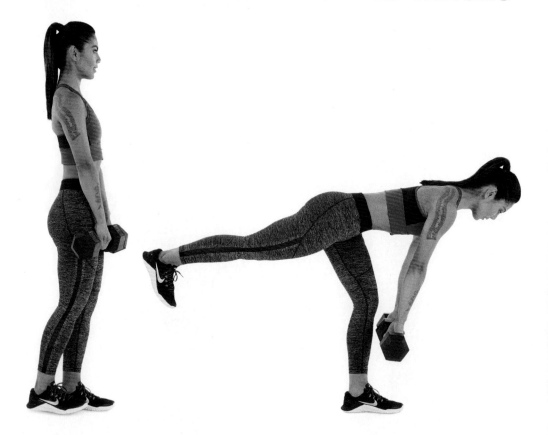

Dumbbell Single-Leg Romanian Deadlift

Stand tall with your feet hip-width apart and hold a pair of dumbbells against your thighs with an overhand grip. Pull your shoulder blades down and together and brace your core. Shift your weight to your left leg and bend your right knee slightly, so that your right foot is hovering off the ground. This is your starting position. Hinge at your hips to lower the weights down the front of your left leg. As you do so, let your right leg lift off the floor behind you. Pause when your torso is parallel to the floor, or you feel a stretch in your hamstrings. Then drive through your left heel and squeeze your glutes to return to the starting position. That's one rep. Complete all reps, then repeat on the opposite side.

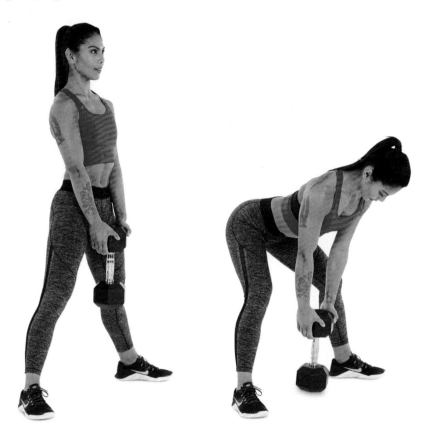

DON'T SQUAT YOUR DEADLIFTS!

Deadlifts involve much less knee flexion (bend) than squats do. During deadlifts, focus on pushing your hips behind you and then thrusting them forward. Keep the knee bend to a minimum!

Dumbbell Sumo Deadlift

Stand tall with your feet about twice shoulder-width apart and hold a dumbbell by the top end with both hands. Maintain a flat back and brace your core. Keeping your back naturally arched, push your hips back and slightly bend your knees to lower the dumbbell until it almost touches the floor or you feel a stretch in your hamstrings. Pause, then drive through your heels and squeeze your glutes to thrust your hips forward to return to a standing position. That's one rep.

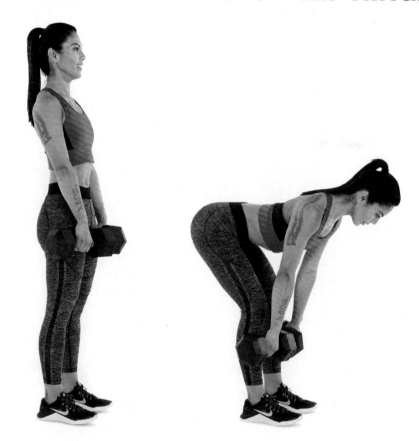

Tempo Dumbbell Romanian Deadlift

Stand tall with your feet hip-width apart and hold a dumbbell in each hand with an overhand grip in front of your hips. Pull your shoulder blades together and brace your core. From here, slowly bend at your hips to lower your torso until it is almost parallel to the floor (or you feel a stretch in your hamstrings). Count to four as you do so. Pause for one second at the bottom of the movement. Drive through your heels and squeeze your glutes to thrust your hips forward and return to a standing position in one second. That's one rep.

(LOWER-)BODY EXERCISES
> HIP ABDUCTIONS

While hip abduction (moving your thigh away from your body) isn't one of the seven basic movement patterns, it's still an important one. Strengthening your hip abductors promotes good form during other lower-body movements and helps to prevent injuries.

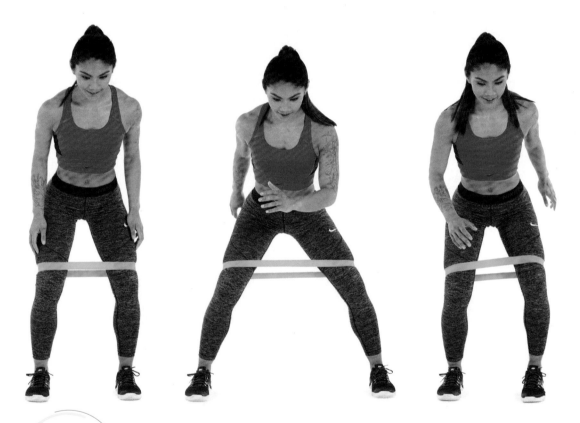

TIGHT ON SPACE?

Perform alternating reps, stepping back and forth in place.

Lateral Band Walk

Loop a miniband around both legs, just above your knees. Stand with your knees bent and feet hip-width apart. From here, step your left foot to the left, then follow with your right, making sure to keep your knees and toes pointed forward the entire time. That's one rep. Complete all reps, then repeat in the opposite direction.

LOWER-BODY EXERCISES
> HIP ABDUCTIONS

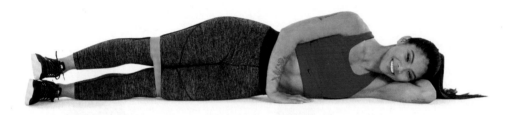

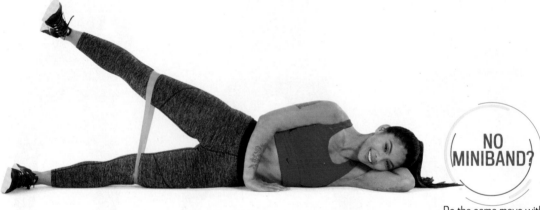

Miniband Side-Lying Hip Abduction

Lie on your left side on the floor with a miniband looped around both legs, just below your knees. Your legs should be straight and stacked. Rest your head on your left arm, and brace your right hand on the floor in front of your belly. From here, without moving any other part of your body, raise your right leg as high as you can. Pause, then lower your leg to return to start. That's one rep. Complete all reps, then repeat on the opposite side.

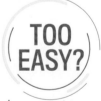

NO MINIBAND?

Do the same move with just your bodyweight, but double the reps.

TOO EASY?

Increase resistance by choosing a "heavier" band.

LOWER-BODY EXERCISES > LUNGES

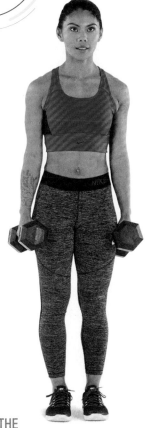

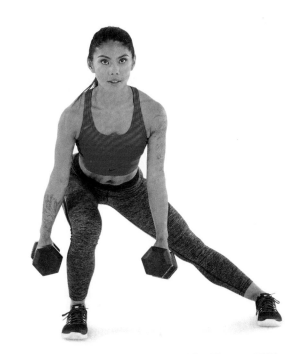

KNOW THE
DIFFERENCE:

LATERAL
LUNGE
VS.
LATERAL
SQUAT

In a lateral lunge, each rep involves stepping one foot to the side and back again. In a lateral squat, your foot never leaves the floor.

Alternating Dumbbell Lateral Lunge

Stand tall with your feet hip-width apart and hold a pair of dumbbells at arm's length next to your sides, your palms facing each other. This is your starting position. From here, take an exaggerated step with your right foot in that direction. Simultaneously push your hips back and bend your right knee to lower your body as far as you can. Pause, then press through your right foot to return to the starting position. Repeat on the opposite side. That's one rep.

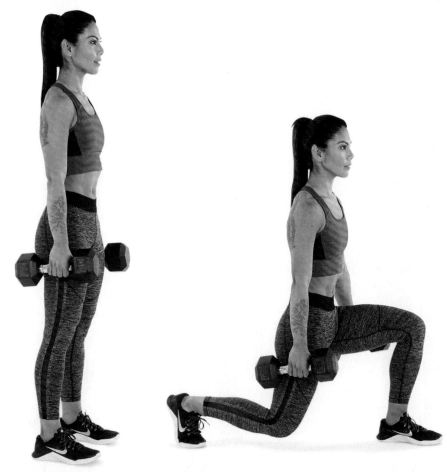

Alternating Dumbbell Reverse Lunge

Holding a pair of dumbbells at your sides, stand tall with your feet hip-width apart. Pull your shoulders back and brace your core. This is your starting position. From here, step backward with your right leg and bend your knees to lower your body toward the floor. Pause, then press through your front foot to return to the starting position. Repeat on the opposite side. That's one rep.

TAKE IT EASY ON YOUR KNEES!

If lunges are uncomfortable on your knees, try angling your torso slightly forward so that the dumbbells lower to the sides of your front foot. This will take some of the stress off of your quads and knees and move it to your glutes.

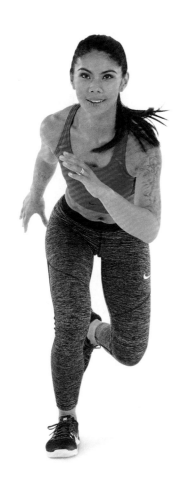
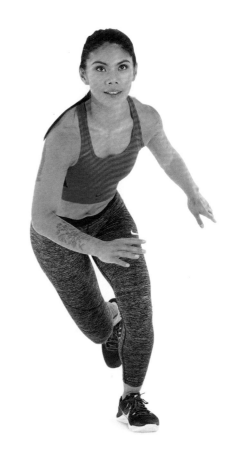

Alternating Lateral Bound

Stand on your right leg with both knees bent and your left foot hovering off the floor. From here, drive through your right foot and swing your arms to jump up and to your left, landing on your left foot with your right foot hovering off the ground. Repeat in the opposite direction. That's one rep.

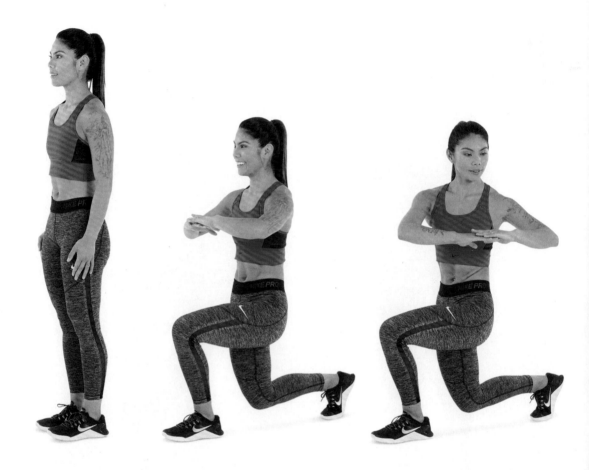

Alternating Reverse Lunge to Twist

Stand tall with your feet hip-width apart. Pull your shoulders back and brace your core. This is your starting position. From here, take a step backward with your right foot, then bend your knees to lower your body toward the floor. Keeping your hips pointed forward, rotate your torso to the left, then reverse to face forward. Pause, then press through your front foot to return to the starting position. Repeat on the opposite side. That's one rep.

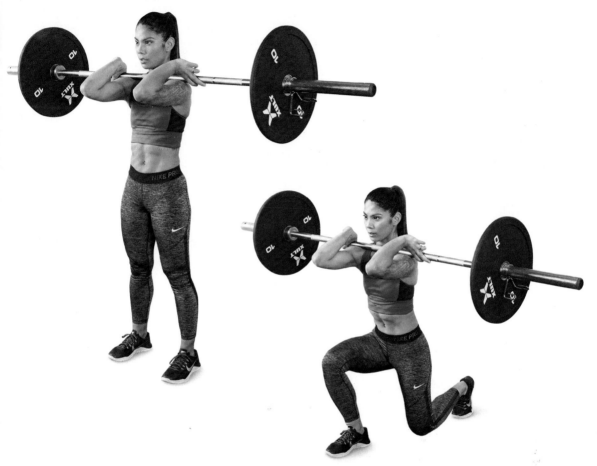

Barbell Reverse Lunge

Stand facing a barbell that's positioned in a squat rack just lower than shoulder height. Grasp the bar with an overhand grip, dip your knees, and let the bar roll back to the tips of your fingers until it rests securely on the front of your shoulders. Raise your upper arms until they're parallel to the floor. (The bar will stay in place as long as you don't allow your elbows to drop as you perform the exercise.) Take a step back and set your feet shoulder-width apart. This is your starting position. Take a step backward with your left foot, then bend your knees to lower your body toward the floor. Pause, then press through your right foot to return to the starting position. That's one rep. Complete all reps and then repeat on the opposite side.

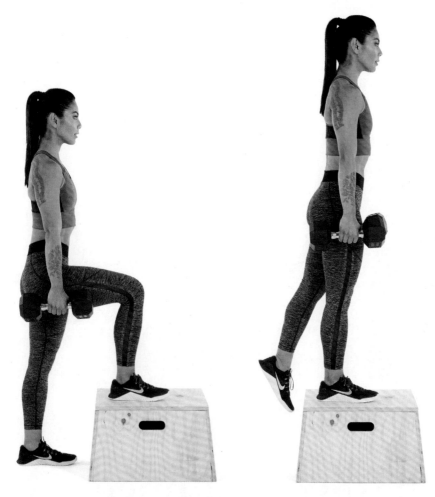

Dumbbell Stepup

Grab a pair of dumbbells and hold them at arm's length at your sides with a neutral grip. Stand in front of a bench or step, and place your right foot firmly on the step. This is your starting position. Drive through your right foot to step up onto the bench, with both legs straight and your left foot hovering. Pause, then slowly bend your right leg to lower to the starting position. That's one rep. Complete all reps, then repeat on the opposite side.

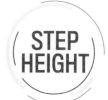

STEP HEIGHT

Choosing a higher or lower step will make the move more or less challenging. Work up to using a step that's high enough that the knee of your lead leg is bent to 90 degrees.

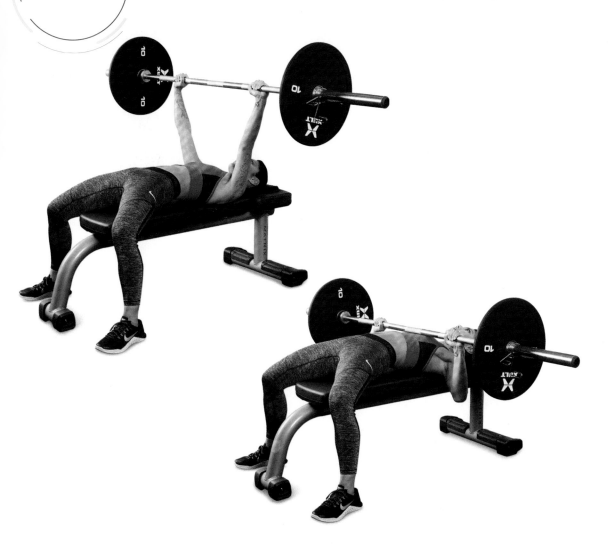

Barbell Bench Press

Lie faceup on a bench. Using an overhand grip that's slightly beyond shoulder width, hold the bar above your sternum with your arms straight. Squeeze your shoulder blades together and lower the bar to your sternum, pulling your elbows toward your sides. Pause, then, keeping your hips in contact with the bench, press the bar back up. That's one rep.

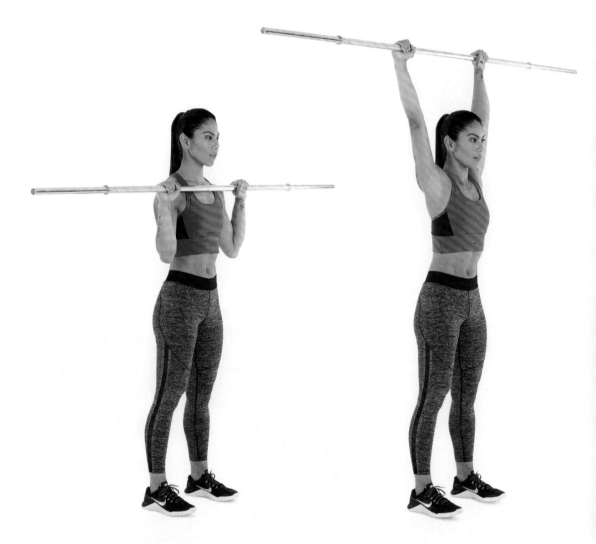

Barbell Overhead Press

Stand tall with your feet shoulder-width apart and knees slightly bent. Hold a barbell at shoulder height in front of your body with an overhand grip that's just wider than shoulder-width apart. Brace your core. From here, press the barbell straight overhead until your arms are straight. Pause, then lower the bar back to start. That's one rep.

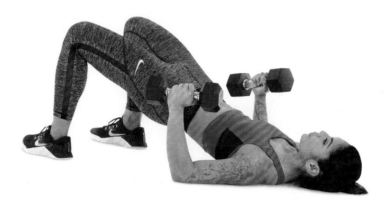

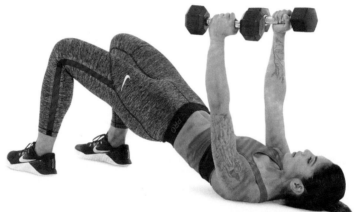

Bridge Hold with Dumbbell Chest Press

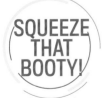

SQUEEZE THAT BOOTY!

Don't let your hips lower to the floor between reps.

Grab a pair of dumbbells and lie faceup on the floor with your knees bent and feet flat on the floor, hip-width apart and about 6 to 8 inches from your glutes. Hold the dumbbells with your palms facing in, your upper arms flat on the floor, and your forearms vertical. Brace your core. Lift your hips so that your body forms a straight line from shoulders to knees. This is your starting position. From here, press the weights directly over your chest until your arms are straight. Pause, then lower the weights to return to the starting position. That's one rep.

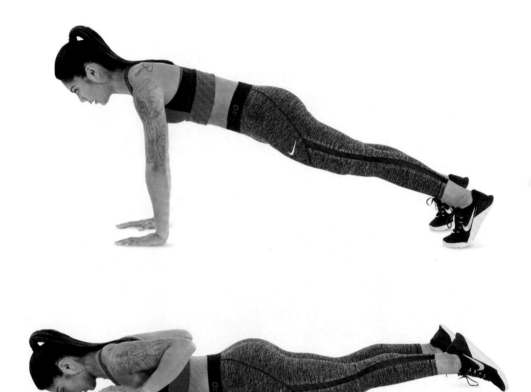

Hand-Release Pushup

Get into a pushup position and place your hands on the floor so that they're slightly wider than your shoulders. Your body should form a straight line from head to heels. Brace your core and pull your shoulders back away from your ears. This is your starting position. From here, bend your elbows to lower your body until your chest rests on the floor. Lift your hands off the floor. Pause, and then push through your hands to return to the starting position. That's one rep.

UPPER-BODY EXERCISES > PUSHES

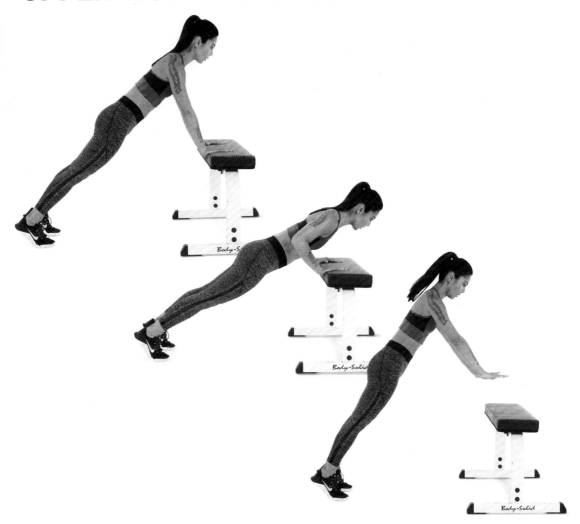

Incline Plyometric Pushup

Get into a pushup position with your hands elevated on a box, step, or bench. Lower your body until your chest nearly touches the bench or other platform. At the bottom of the move, drive forcefully through your chest and arms so that you "explode" up and your hands leave the platform. That's one rep. As your hands land back on the surface, bend your elbows to cushion the impact and lower your body into the next rep.

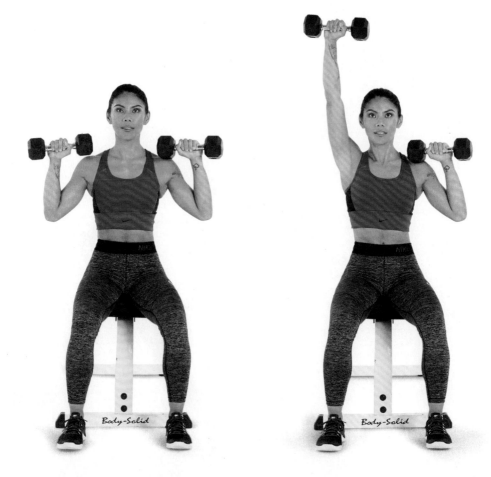

Seated Alternating Overhead Press

Sit on a bench with your torso upright, holding a pair of dumbbells just outside of your shoulders with an overhand grip and your elbows bent and pointed to the floor. Brace your core. From here, press one weight up until your arm is straight. Pause, then lower the dumbbell back to start. Repeat on the opposite side. That's one rep.

UPPER-BODY EXERCISES > PUSHES

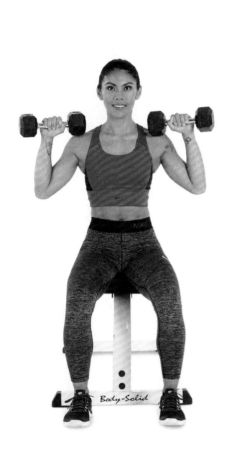
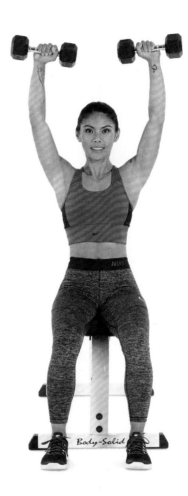

Seated Dumbbell Overhead Press

Sit on a bench with your torso upright. Hold a pair of dumbbells just outside your shoulders with an overhand grip and your elbows bent and pointed to the floor. Brace your core. From here, press the dumbbells up until your arms are straight. Pause, then lower the dumbbells back to start. That's one rep.

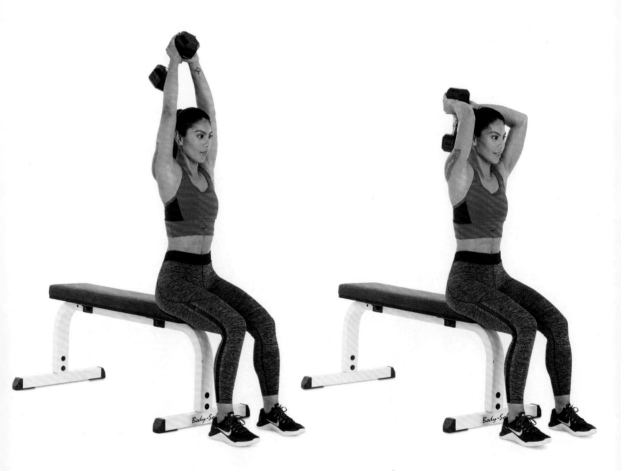

Seated Overhead Triceps Extension

Sit on a bench with your torso upright. Hold a dumbbell straight above your head, with both hands cupping the top end of the weight. Brace your core. From here, bend your elbows to lower the weight behind your head as far as you comfortably can. Pause, then, keeping your elbows tucked in close to your head and upper arms vertical, press the weight up to return to start. That's one rep.

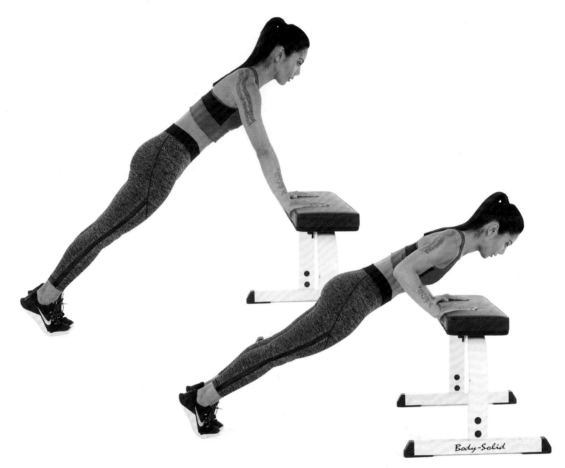

Tempo Incline Pushup

Get into a pushup position with your hands elevated on a box, step, bench, or fixed barbell on a squat rack. This reduces the amount of your bodyweight you have to lift, making the exercise easier. Your hands should be slightly wider than your shoulders, and your body should form a straight line from head to heels. Brace your core. From here, lower your body slowly over the course of four seconds until your chest nearly touches the bench (or whatever platform you're using), pulling your elbows in toward your sides. Pause for one second at the bottom, and then push through your hands to return to start in one second. That's one rep. Increase the incline to lessen the resistance. Decrease the incline to make the move more challenging.

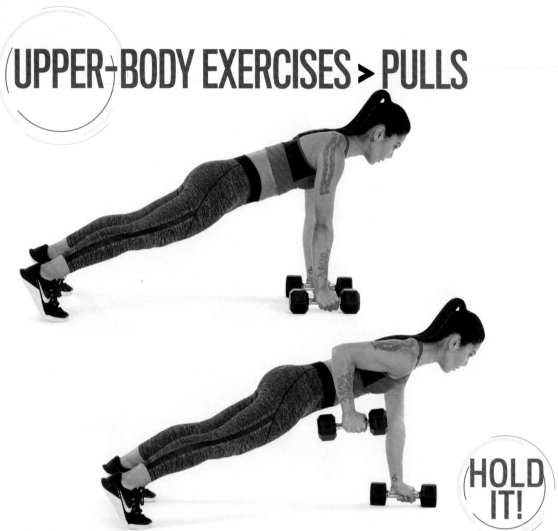

Alternating Plank Row

Grab a pair of hex dumbbells and get down into a pushup position on the floor. Place the dumbbells so that your hands are just wider than shoulder-width apart, your palms facing each other. Your body should form a straight line from head to heels. Brace your core and pull your shoulders back away from your ears. From here, bend your right elbow and pull the weight up to your side, keeping your elbow tucked in by your torso. Pause, then lower the weight down to start. Repeat on the opposite side. That's one rep.

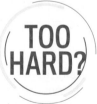

HOLD IT!

Your torso should not rotate as you row.

TOO HARD?

Lower the amount of weight used, rather than dropping to your knees.

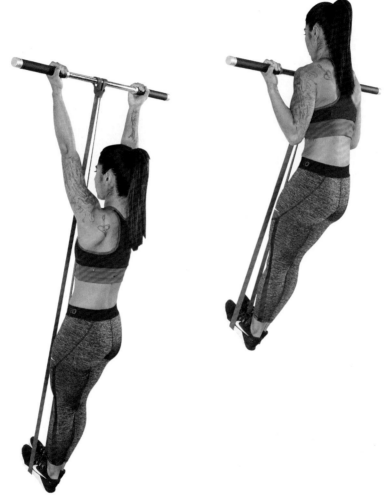

Band-Assisted Chinup

Tie a large looped resistance band around a pullup bar and grab the bar with an under-hand grip that's just wider than shoulder-width apart. Place one foot in the sling created by the band. Brace your core and hang at arm's length. Squeeze your shoulder blades down and together. This is your starting position. From here, pull through your arms to raise your collarbones to the bar. Pause, then reverse the movement to return to the start-ing position. That's one rep.

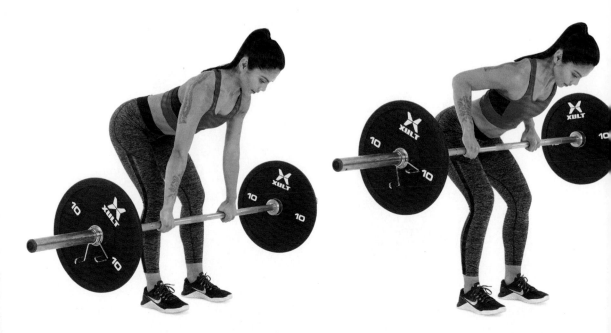

Barbell Bent-Over Row

Stand tall with your feet hip-width apart and hold a barbell with an overhand grip, your hands just wider than shoulder-width apart. Push your hips back and bend your knees to lower your torso until it's almost parallel to the floor. Brace your core. This is your starting position. From here, squeeze your shoulder blades back and together, bend your elbows, and pull the barbell to your torso. Pause, then slowly reverse the movement to return to the starting position. That's one rep.

MIRROR, MIRROR

Fight the temptation to watch your form in the weight-room mirror! It's important to keep your neck in line with the rest of your spine during all exercises. During bent-over rows, that means you should look at the floor a few feet in front of you. Look up, and you unwittingly dump the weight into your lower back.

UPPER-BODY EXERCISES > PULLS

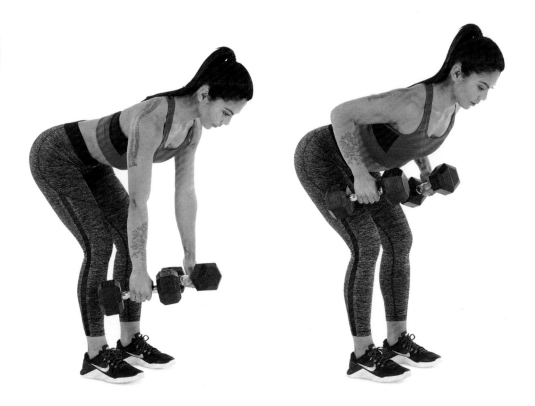

Dumbbell Bent-Over Row

Stand tall with your feet hip-width apart and hold a dumbbell in each hand, palms facing each other. Push your hips back and bend your knees to lower your torso until it's almost parallel to the floor. Brace your core. This is your starting position. From here, squeeze your shoulder blades back and together, bend your elbows, and pull the weights to your torso. Pause, then reverse the movement to return to the starting position. That's one rep.

UPPER-BODY EXERCISES > PULLS

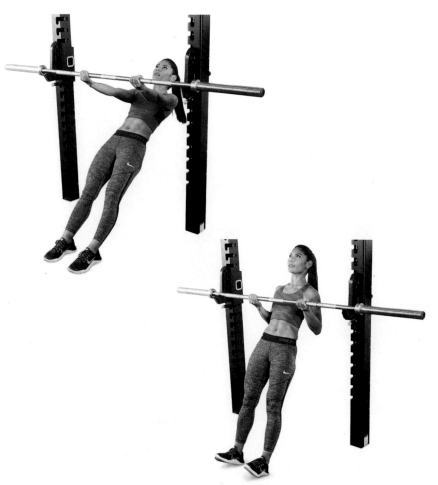

A WORD ON INCLINE

To reduce the percentage of your bodyweight that you have to row, increase the incline by raising the barbell. This will work your upper back to a higher degree. Lowering the barbell will up the amount of weight you have to row as well as increase recruitment of your lats in your mid-back.

OPTIONS, OPTIONS

You can either use a squat rack or Smith machine to do the exercise, or, if they're available, TRX straps. Because TRX straps introduce instability, you will be able to row less weight (meaning you'll need more of an incline) with the straps than you will with a fixed barbell.

Inverted Row

Grab a fixed barbell with an underhand grip, your hands just wider than shoulder-width apart. Hang with your arms straight and your feet out in front of you, so that your body forms a straight line from head to heels. Brace your core. This is your starting position. From here, squeeze your shoulder blades back and together, bend your elbows, and pull your chest to the bar. Pause, then lower your body to the starting position. That's one rep.

UPPER-BODY EXERCISES > PULLS

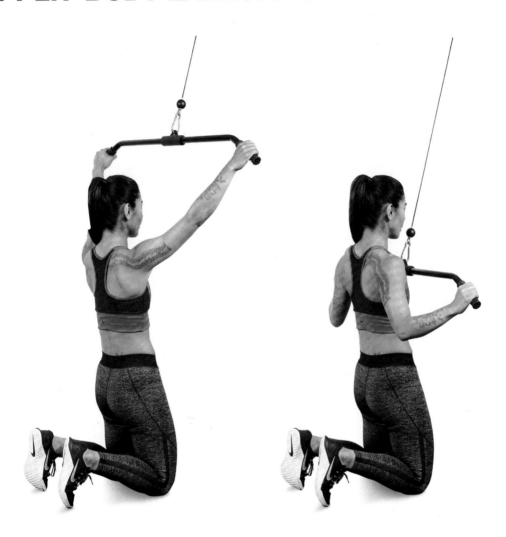

Kneeling Lat Pulldown

Kneel on both knees facing a cable machine with a lat bar attached to a high setting. Grab the bar with an overhand grip and brace your core. From here, squeeze your shoulder blades down and together, bend your elbows, and pull the bar to your collarbones. Pause, then reverse the movement to return to start. That's one rep.

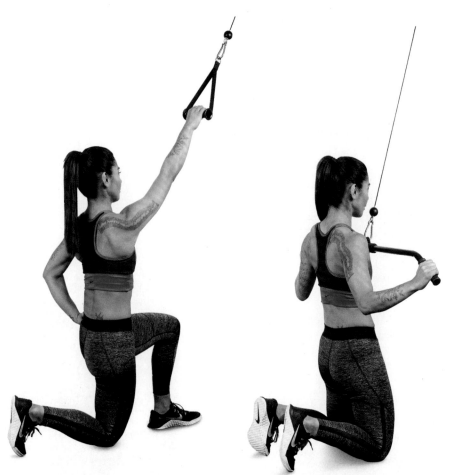

Single-Arm Half-Kneeling Lat Pulldown

Kneel on your right knee facing a cable machine, and, with your right hand, grab a stirrup handle attached to a high setting. Brace your core. From here, squeeze your shoulder blade back and down, bend your elbow, and pull the handle to the side of your chest. Pause, then reverse the movement to return to start. That's one rep. Complete all reps, then repeat on the opposite side.

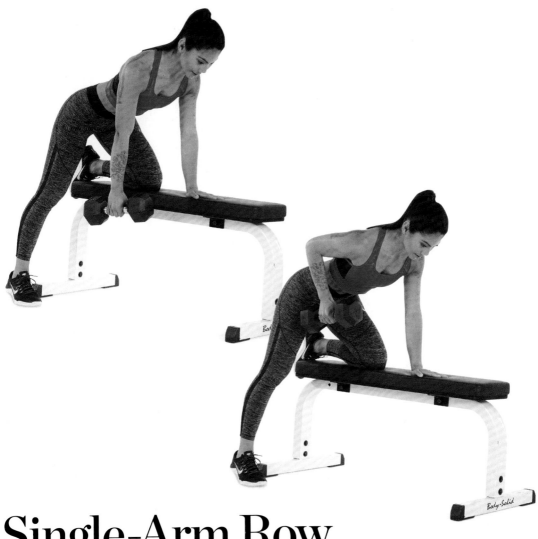

Single-Arm Row

Grab a dumbbell in your right hand and place your left hand and left knee on a bench. Let the dumbbell hang at arm's length, palm facing in, and brace your core. This is your starting position. From here, pull the dumbbell to the side of your torso, keeping your elbow tucked in close to your side. Pause, then lower the dumbbell to return to the starting position. That's one rep. Complete all reps, then repeat on the opposite side.

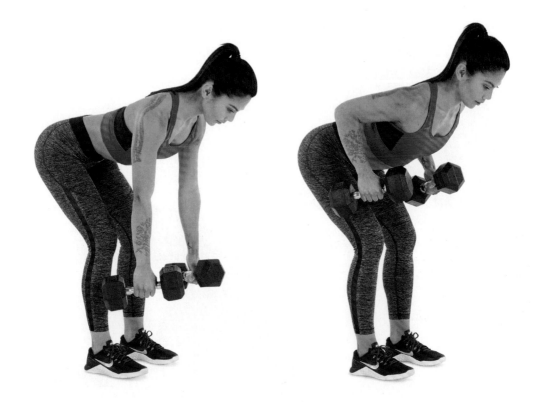

Tempo Dumbbell Bent-Over Row

Stand tall with your feet hip-width apart and hold a dumbbell in each hand, your palms facing each other. Push your hips back and bend your knees to lower your torso until it's almost parallel to the floor. Brace your core. This is your starting position. From here, squeeze your shoulder blades back and together, bend your elbows, and pull the weights to your torso in one second. Pause for one second, then slowly reverse the movement to return to the starting position over the course of four seconds. That's one rep.

UPPER-BODY EXERCISES > PULLS

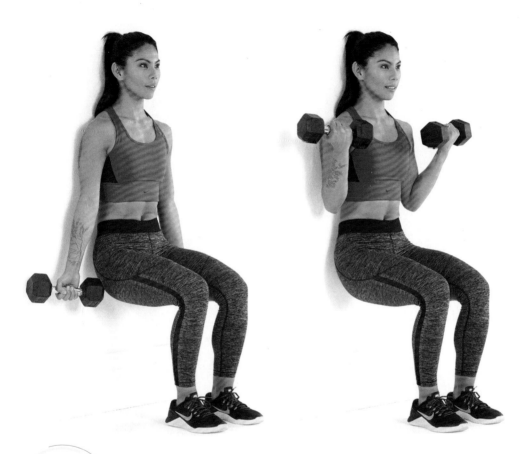

GET LOW!

Try to get your thighs parallel to the floor. Keep in mind that the lower you "sit," the farther your feet will need to be from the wall.

Wall-Sit Biceps Curl

Stand tall with your feet hip-width apart and your back facing a wall about 12 to 18 inches behind you. Hold a pair of dumbbells with an underhand grip at your sides. From here, push your hips back and bend your knees to "sit" with your back flat against the wall. This is your starting position. Holding the seated position, curl both weights up to your shoulders. Pause, then lower the weights to return to the starting position. That's one rep.

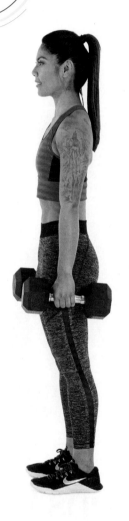 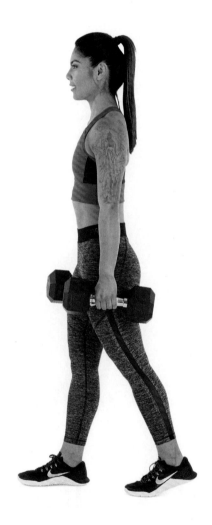

Farmer's Carry

Grab a pair of heavy dumbbells and hold them at your sides with your palms facing in. Brace your core. From here, slowly walk forward, imagining that a string attached to the top of your head is pulling your torso straight and tall. Each step is one rep.

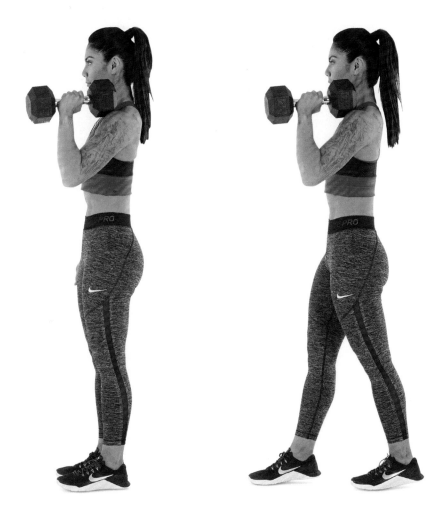

Rack-Position Carry

Stand tall and hold a dumbbell in your left hand at your shoulder with your palm facing in and your elbow pointed toward the floor. Brace your core. From here, slowly walk forward, imagining that a string attached to the top of your head is pulling your torso straight and tall. Don't let yourself lean to one side. Each step is one rep. Complete all reps, then repeat on the opposite side.

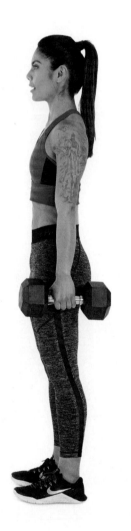
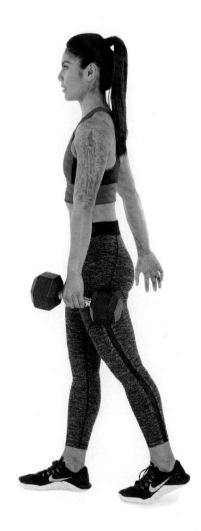

Suitcase Carry

Grab a heavy dumbbell and hold it at your side with your palm facing in. Brace your core. From here, slowly walk forward, imagining that a string attached to the top of your head is pulling your torso straight and tall. Don't let yourself lean to one side. Each step is one rep. Complete all reps, then repeat on the opposite side.

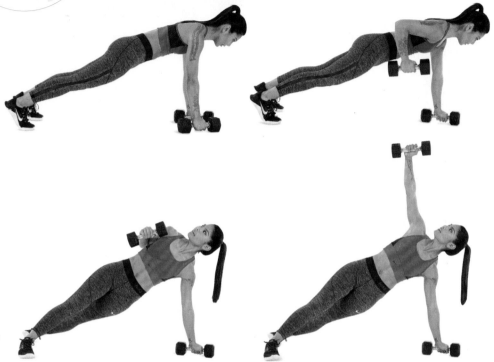

Plank Row Rotation and Extension

Grab a pair of hex dumbbells and get down into a pushup position on the floor. Place the dumbbells so that your hands are just wider than shoulder-width apart, your palms facing each other. Your body should form a straight line from head to heels. Brace your core and pull your shoulders back away from your ears. From here, bend your right elbow and pull the weight up to your side, keeping your elbow tucked in by your torso. Pause, then rotate your hips to the right to get into a side plank on your left arm, then straighten your right arm toward the ceiling. Pause, then reverse the movement to return to the starting position. Repeat on the opposite side. That's one rep.

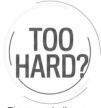

TOO HARD?

This is a challenging move, so make sure to use a light weight.

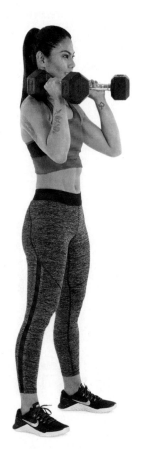

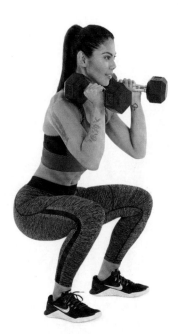

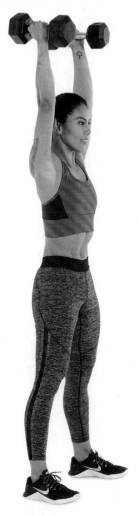

Squat and Overhead Press

Stand tall with your feet shoulder-width apart and hold a pair of dumbbells in front of your shoulders, your elbows pointed down and palms facing each other. Pull your shoulders back and brace your core. This is your starting position. Push your hips back and bend your knees to lower your body until your thighs are parallel to the floor (or as far as you can comfortably go). Pause, then push through your heels to return to standing, while simultaneously pressing the dumbbells overhead until your arms are straight. Lower the weights back to the starting position. That's one rep.